The Smart Couple's Guide to Getting Pregnant, An Integrated Approach

The Smart Couple's Guide to Getting Pregnant, An Integrated Approach

Dr. Farrar Duro, DOM, FABORM

Revised Edition, 2017

First Printing, 2015

Florida Complete Wellness, Inc 4745 Volunteer Rd, Ste 304 Southwest Ranches, FL 33330 www.FloridaCompleteWellness.com

Disclaimer: The contents of this book are for informational purposes only and are NOT a substitute for professional medical advice, diagnosis, treatment or substitute for a formal medical consultation. Always seek the advice of your physician or other qualified health provider with any questions you may have regarding a medical condition. You should always consult your physician regarding the specifics of your case. Nothing contained in this book, including the questions and answers written, is intended to be medical advice, diagnosis or treatment.

Acknowledgements

I would like to thank my teachers for inspiring me to write this guide. You've come into my life as my patients, doctors, professors, family and friends who have shared the same passion for shedding more light on infertility. I would also like to express my deepest gratitude to the doctors and staff at IVF Florida, UHealth Fertility at the University of Miami, and IVFMD. Thank you to Dr. Lin Chai, along with Dr. Paul Magarelli and Diane Cridennda for your tireless research and contributions to TCM and reproductive medicine. Dr. Marion Colas-Lacombe, I am grateful for your openness to answering my OBGYN questions throughout the years. I am also humbled and grateful for the lessons that my patients have taught me over the last 15 years and apply them daily to my practice. I am also thankful to Stephanie, Colleen, Marilyn and Kim at Florida Complete Wellness-my family away from home.

To my husband Joaquin, you never cease to inspire me with your support and admiration. For my children, Dailey and Sebastian and my stepsons Marcos and Sebas...thank you for bringing me joy every day. And Mom, thank you for listening. You will finally stop hearing me whine about not having enough hours in the day to finish this book.

Introduction

As a licensed acupuncture physician certified by the American Board of Oriental Reproductive Medicine, I have treated hundreds of couples undergoing assisted reproductive techniques over the past 15 years with acupuncture and Traditional Chinese medicine. Navigating the rough waters of infertility can prove to be extremely frustrating, so I created this guide for couples like you who want to make the most informed decisions on questions that may not be answered in a typical fertility clinic or gynecological setting.

By reading this book you have taken an exciting step in gaining control of your fertility treatment and better understanding your treatment. Please share it with your providers so that their knowledge of your specific case may be deepened and enriched. You just may stand out as the most organized fertility patient that they've seen all year! Often your current medical team may not be familiar with the type of research available on acupuncture and reproductive medicine in this book, so use it to your advantage!

Experience has shown that by having a clear plan and understanding what your reproductive endocrinologist, nutritionist, psychologist, gynecologist, acupuncturist, etc. have in mind can lead to shorter, more effective treatment. In the end, we all want what you want- a healthy mom and baby with as few complications as possible. It is the aim of this book to provide clarity and reassurance to you, whether you have been struggling with infertility for nine months or nine years. If this book saves you from one more month of waiting for a child, then its purpose has been fulfilled.

Baby dust and best of luck in the journey ahead,

Farrar Duro, DOM, FABORM

Contents

Chapter One-Why Can't We Conceive?

Danny and Ana had been trying unsuccessfully for two years to get pregnant. Every night, after Danny fell asleep Ana would venture into the fertility chat rooms just in case she missed something posted the day before. Her supplement regimen was a long list of suggestions from her fertility forum friends that filled a large pill organizer. "I'm too young to have to take this many pills," she thought. "If only Danny would step up and just take his multivitamin, I wouldn't feel like I was doing this alone."

It didn't help matters that Ana's best friend was now four months pregnant, and told her to "just relax and it will happen" whenever Ana expressed her frustration. Now Ana's new fertility acupuncturist was suggesting she speak to her gynecologist about getting a referral to an IVF clinic so she and her husband could start all the necessary tests. What if her new fertility doctor didn't approve of her acupuncture treatments or supplement use? Would her husband be on board with going to a few consultations with different clinics to make sure their new doctor was a good fit? Ana's stress level had climbed to Mount Everest proportions and she needed some clear answers. She vowed to stay away from the chat rooms for the next few weeks and start putting her fertility plan in action.

If you are one of the estimated 6.1 million couples in America who are having problems conceiving, it's comforting to know what options are available. Finding out the cause of infertility can be time-consuming and expensive, so the goal should be to narrow down the diagnosis quickly. With proper treatment, the good news is that two out of three couples will be successful in having a baby, and the earlier that treatment is sought the better. The concept of regulating the menstrual cycle to promote fertility has been strongly emphasized for centuries in Eastern medicine. In the Song dynasty (960-1279 CE), a doctor named Chén Zì-Míng claimed that "menstruation must be regulated first, if not, myriad illnesses may ensue; if menstruation is regular, the woman will get pregnant."

What Is Infertility?

Infertility is defined as the inability of couples of reproductive age to establish a pregnancy within one year through unprotected intercourse. The basic causes of infertility are as follows: 50% female, 35% male, 10% unexplained, and 5% other causes. When we are in our mother's womb at 20 weeks gestation, our ovaries contain about 6-7 million oocytes (eggs), which decline to 1-2 million by the time we're born. By puberty, there are only 300,000-400,000 follicles remaining in the ovaries. Of those, only about 400 eggs are ovulated in a lifetime until roughly age 51 when menopause occurs.

The Brain's Role in Hormone Production

To understand the process of reproduction and how treatments such as acupuncture and mind-body techniques come into play, it's important to look at the brain. One area of the brain called the anterior pituitary is responsible for the production of the hormones LH (luteinizing hormone) and FSH (follicle stimulating hormone), which act on the ovaries. Gonadotropin Releasing Hormone (GNRH) is released by the hypothalamus and acts on the pituitary in coordinated pulse frequencies. The other hormones that you may be familiar with, estrogen (E2) and progesterone (P4) act on the endometrium (uterine lining) and are produced by the growing follicle and corpus luteum. During pregnancy, the placenta assumes production of progesterone at about 10-12 weeks. This is often the time your reproductive specialist will tell you to stop any progesterone supplementation after an IVF cycle.

During a normal menstrual cycle, progesterone and estrogen contribute to thickening the lining to allow for implantation. Just before your menses occurs, estrogen and progesterone drop to allow for proper shedding of the endometrium. Chinese herbal treatment can also help regulate your menses by working with the distinct phases of the cycle. For example, one of the formulas we use in our clinic is called Blossom by Evergreen Herbs. Blossom is comprised of four herbal formulas, one for each week of the month beginning with Phase One during the menstrual cycle and ending with Phase Four. A course of herbal treatment is often recommended prior to or along with acupuncture for at least 3-6 months when preparing for a medicated fertility cycle or can be used as a stand alone treatment in the case of unexplained infertility. Once fertility medications are commenced, Chinese herbal medicine may be discontinued at the discretion of the treating reproductive specialist and Traditional Chinese Medicine practitioner so as not to interfere with proper medication dosage.

Chapter Two-Getting To Know You

In our clinic, the number one question we get from patients is "How do I know when I'm ovulating?" Ways of monitoring ovulation are too numerous to list, but a search of ovulation predictors online will give you some idea.

I often ask women to combine basal body temperature (BBT) charting with a reliable ovulation predictor test for no more than two or three months to determine if ovulation is occurring. Charting your temperatures is free, and aside from being a minor hassle, you can gleam important information that can be useful for you and your fertility specialists.

Knowing your own body and being able to tell when you are fertile or ovulating has its benefits. There are only certain times during your menstrual cycle when you are fertile or can get pregnant, so it pays to know when those times are.

Your body will give you clear clues and signals as to when your fertile window is approaching. A woman is fertile when she is ovulating and for about four to five days before ovulation when fertile cervical mucus is present.

The Big O

Ovulation usually occurs mid-cycle. More precisely, ovulation usually occurs fourteen days before the onset of bleeding. However, ovulation can be delayed by many factors, including sickness, alcohol or prescription drug intake, travel, and stress. This is the main reason why simply counting the days can be inaccurate. To make matters even more confusing, a study published in the British Medical Journal in

2000 concluded in only about 30% of women is the fertile window entirely within the days of the menstrual cycle identified by clinical guidelines—that is, between days 10 and 17. You will find your success in tracking your fertility will be far greater when you become attune to your own personal fertility signals rather than just counting the days.

It is a brief guide that I have put together from both personal and patient comments throughout the years. The time frame varies; so don't worry if your cycle is not the same. Keep in mind that each woman's physiology is different.

Steps to Recognizing Fertility Signs:

-Find a system of recording your menstrual cycle and fertile times that is easy for you to use. Using this book or your normal diary or calendar works just as well as long as you remember to write down the information you need. A plethora of free smart phone applications exist and make charting even easier.

-Use your system regularly.

-Start observing your mucus, and keep a record...write it down. This book offers a blank charting template, along with instructions that you may copy and use each month. Alternately, use a website such as FertilityFriend.com or similar smart phone apps as many of our patients do. This offers convenience and has the added benefit of being shared via email to your practitioner.

Week 1 (Menses)

The menstrual cycle begins on the first day of full flow, not spotting. At this point, you may note any cramps, clots or mucus-like discharge visible on your pad or tampon. At our clinic we recommend using pads since they are more like a canvas on which the quality of your menstrual blood is best viewed. We ask our patients to note color as well, the best being a bright red flow lasting at least 4 days and the worse scenario being dark brown-to-black large clots.

Typically, after the menses there is an increase in physical energy and vitality. Emotionally, your mood is more outgoing and sociable. Sleep patterns and appetite return to normal and vaginal mucus is dry or absent.

Week 2 (Post-menses): As ovulation approaches mucus becomes more wet, slip- prey, white (whatever is your individual pattern.) Note cervical mucus changes as well as any unusual spotting or cramping. In Traditional Chinese Medicine, we refer to this stage as the Yin building into Yang.

Ovulation/Day 14 approximately*

Mucus is very wet and slippery, easily allowing penetration of sperm. Breasts may be tender, and mood swings, increase in libido, cramps, and desire to be with your partner may occur more strongly. At this point, note any positive surges on the LH sticks or fertility monitor and watch for your temperature to drop and then spike from 0.3-1 degree.

Week 3-Post-ovulation and beginning of premenstrual phase

Mucus production slows, becomes drier and thicker. Moods balance out again.

Week 4-Premenstrual phase

Premenstrual symptoms kick in, which can range from bloating, cramps, head- aches, mood swings, food cravings, and insomnia. This temperature rise should continue until your period comes, or if it's your lucky month it will continue to rise further past 16-18 days after ovulation. This is a strong clue to take a home pregnancy test! Often we see a pronounced three-step rise on the BBT chart associated with a positive pregnancy test. If the temperatures drop, this is associated also with a drop in estrogen and decreased energy levels along with libido.

** Please note that ovulation may not always occur at day fourteen, which is why counting the days or the rhythm method is an unreliable and often incorrect method of gauging fertility. However, periods do usually arrive fourteen days after ovulation. In irregular cycles, it is the first half of the cycle or follicular phase which varies in length (rather than the second half of the cycle), as bleeding almost always occurs twelve to fourteen days after ovulation unless there is a progesterone deficiency or luteal phase defect (LPD).

It is only through getting to know your individual cycle that you can know what your pattern is. If you experience a constant reliable rhythm - then that rhythm is yours, regardless of how it fits into the 'norm'.

What's with the Mucus?

Cervical Mucus is one of the most important indicators of fertility. It will change throughout the menstrual cycle from being dry, thick or pasty (infertile) to being wet and slippery (fertile). It is the job of the cervical mucus to either restrict or allow sperm penetration through the cervix. Often, it may be difficult to discern whether or not you have any fertile mucus, but a quick glance at the underwear lining can sometimes be of help. Some women have noted that they have to wipe a little more when urinating or even think they might have a vaginal infection if it's very plentiful. Each woman varies in the amount of cervical mucus she produces, and this can even vary from cycle to cycle depending on fluctuating hormone levels.

Observing cervical mucus becomes simple with a little practice. You are only interested in the mucus that is readily observable at the mouth of the vagina. You need only touch the mouth of the vagina (no need to touch inside), the outside of the opening or alternatively wipe the vaginal mouth with a tissue and feel mucus from that.

Dry or none = infertile

Wet, profuse and slippery = fertile

The changes from dry to wet indicate that fertile phase is coming and changes from wet to dry indicate fertility is lessening.

We have found that your peak fertility day is usually the day of the most fertile cervical mucus discharge. As sperm can live for up to 3-4 days in fertile mucus, the window of time you have to conceive can be as long as five days prior to ovulation. For instance, I've seen several instances of a patient appearing disheartened due to their perceived "bad timing" prior to their partner going out of town, only to have happy news at the end of the month. And no, the partner did not request a DNA test!

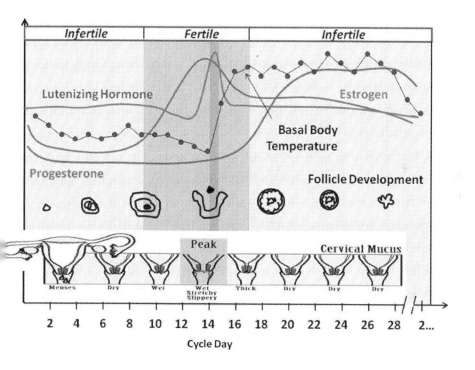

(Image courtesy of http://wvmarriage.org)

Charting your Basal Body Temperature (BBT)

Charting your BBTs is really pretty easy. Basically, what you are doing is taking your temperature first thing each day and plotting the temperature on a chart.
What you are looking for is to see a shift of at least .4 degrees Fahrenheit after ovulation making your chart biphasic (showing low temperatures before ovulation in
the follicular phase, and higher ones after ovulation in the luteal phase). Be sure to ovulation tests (urine LH strips) in conjunction with your basal charting to provide you with an accurate sense of your most fertile time of month. Take your temperature first thing in the morning before you get out of bed or even speak -- leave your thermometer at your bedside within easy reach so you don't have to move much to get it. If you use a glass thermometer, make sure you shake it down before going to bed.

Try to take the temperature at as close to the same time each day as possible -- set an alarm if you need to. Staying within a half hour either side of your average time is a good idea because your temp can vary with the time (i.e., if you usually take your temperature at 6 a.m., it is OK to take your BBT between 5:30-6:30, but the closer to 6 the better). The normal variation is by up to .2 degrees per hour -- lower if you take your temperature early, higher if you take it late. It is best to take your BBT after a minimum of 5 hours sleep, and at least 3 in a row is preferable. You can take your temperature orally, vaginally, or rectally --just stay with the same method for the entire cycle and try to place the thermometer the same way each day (same location of your mouth, same depth vaginally and rectally). Plot your temperature on your chart each day, but refrain from reading too much into it until the cycle is done. Some women, not all, have a temperature drop when they ovulate. If you see your temperature drop, it is a good idea to have sex in case you are ovulating. What you are looking for is a temperature shift of at least .4 degrees over a 48- hour period to indicate ovulation.

This shift should be above the highest temperatures in the previous six days, allowing one temperature to be thrown out as inaccurate (fluke, illness). Perhaps the best way to explain this is to show an example.

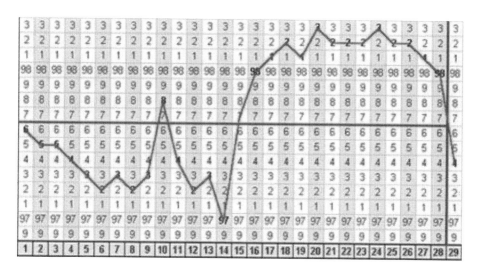

In the image above, the seven BBTs before ovulation are 97.2, 97.3, 97.8, 97.4, 97.2, 97.3, 97.0 then it jumps to 97.7 and then 98. Ovulation most likely occurred on the day with the 97.0 and you can comfortably draw a cover line at 97.6. You just ignore the 97.8 on day 10. After you see a temperature shift for at least three days, or at the end of your cycle, you can draw a cover line between your follicular phase and luteal phase temperatures. With luck, it is easy to see a clear shift and draw your line between the highest follicular phase BBT and the lowest luteal phase BBT as in the sample above. The main reason for drawing this line is just to clearly delineate that your chart is biphasic.

Look at the chart at the end of the month to analyze what happened. Chart for a few months and look for patterns. If your temperature stays up for 18 days or more after ovulation, you should test for pregnancy. One thing to note is that women with ovulatory cycles but with irregular cycle lengths, the greatest variation from cycle to cycle should be in the follicular phase. The luteal phase should be relatively constant (within 1-2 days). So if one has a cycle that ranges from 28-34 days, and a luteal phase of 14 days, ovulation would occur somewhere between days 14-20 -- not the middle of a cycle, not day 14. This is the biggest mistake women with long cycles make when trying to conceive.

Charting Cervical Mucus and Cervical Position

If you want a clearer picture of your cycle, it is best to combine charting your BBT with charting your cervical mucus (CM) and perhaps also charting your cervical position.

There are several ways to chart your mucus, and you have to find the approach that is best for you. You can simply examine your toilet tissue after wiping. You will see more mucus after you have a bowel movement. Another way is to insert two fingers and gently take a little pinch of mucus from the cervix. The easiest positions for most women would be sitting on the toilet, one foot up on the toilet or bathtub, or squatting. If you have trouble reaching, you can ask your partner to check for you. For most, the best position to do this would be for the woman to get on all fours on the bed, or chest down on a pillow, and let the partner insert fingers from behind. Otherwise your partner will be crawling around on the floor!

Cervical mucus varies from dry, to sticky, to creamy, to egg-white (EW) before ovulation in most women. Note that there is now a product on the market for trying-to-conceive women, Fertile CM, that is designed to help encourage the production of abundant "fertile-quality" cervical mucus.

FREQUENTLY ASKED BBT QUESTIONS

Basal Body Temperature Questions Q: What will my BBT chart tell me?

A: The goal is to find out if you are ovulating and help you time intercourse. If you see a definite biphasic chart, that's a good sign. You can also tell whether your luteal phase is long enough if your temperatures are up for at least 12 days after ovulation.

Q: How long should my temperature stay up after ovulation?

Ideally, 14 days. Some doctors say anything over 10 days is acceptable, but it really makes sense to test for luteal phase defect if one typically shows 12 days or less of high temperatures. You can test for luteal phase defect with a serum progesterone level and/or an endometrial biopsy. Many doctors will want to see two cycles of low progesterone or out of phase biopsies before making a definite luteal phase defect diagnosis.

Q: My temperature dropped for a day in the luteal phase, does that mean this cycle is a bust?
A: Not unless it stays down. Some people have a short drop that may go well be- low the cover line that is a secondary estrogen surge (which may be accompanied by mucus). Q: How long should I chart before seeing a doctor if I suspect infertility?

A: Good question! If your cycles are irregular, you shouldn't waste time on BBTs alone -- see a doctor and find out what may be causing the irregularity. If you do have normal-length cycles and decide to start charting, you only need to wait about 3 months to establish a problem and seek help. For example, if you have a 28-day cycle, but ovulate on day 18, and that happens 2-3 months in a row, you should see your doctor. Otherwise it depends on your age and urgency. It's not a bad idea for everyone to get preconception advice and blood work yearly when considering trying to conceive.

Q: What are average BBTs?

A: The average range of BBTs is between 97.0-97.7 before ovulation and 97.7-99.0 after ovulation. Ideally, a woman's temperature will not bounce around more than .5 degrees in the follicular phase and will stay above the cover line during the luteal phase.

Q: My BBTs are lower/higher than average, what does this mean?

A: Either case warrants checking your thyroid. Low BBTs are often a sign of hypothyroidism, which can cause some fertility and pregnancy problems. Excessively high temperatures may indicate hyperthyroidism.

Q: I did an ovulation predictor kit, how long after the positive should my BBT rise?

A: You should ovulate 12-48 hours after the positive ovulation predictor test, and your BBTs should go up within 48 hours of ovulating. It can take up to 4-5 days to see the rise, but ideally you see it within 3 days.

Q: My chart looks more like the Rocky Mountains than anything else, what does that mean?

A: Most likely a) you are not taking your BBTs consistently or sleep erratically, b) you are taking your BBTs orally and you sleep with your mouth open, or c) you are not ovulating. If being more consistent, or switching to taking your BBTs vaginally or rectally, doesn't help, you should go to the doctor to have your hormone levels checked out and see what may be causing your lack of ovulation.

Q: How late in a cycle can one ovulate?

A: It is possible to ovulate very late in a cycle -- there is not any day limit -- so a long cycle doesn't mean there is no hope. Long cycles do, however, reduce opportunities to get pregnant and warrant looking into. It is also a good idea to have at least one cycle every 3 months, brought on by medication if needed, so that the uterine lining does not become too thick.

Q: Can I tell I am pregnant from a BBT chart?

A: You are most likely pregnant if your BBTs stay up for 18 or more days after ovulation. It is also common to see a triphasic chart, a second shift sometime during the luteal phase, when pregnancy is achieved.

Q: Do I really need BBT thermometer, or will a fever thermometer do?

A: A BBT thermometer is more reliable and more accurate. You really need it to be accurate to .1 degrees. The main plus of the digital BBT over a fever BBT thermometer is speed. The BBT digital is more accurate for some people, and it only takes 30-60 seconds, which can matter if you are waiting to go to the bathroom first thing in the morning. The digital ones are harder to break and remember the temperature for you if you don't want to chart it immediately.

Q: Are my BBTs as accurate if I am taking fertility medications such as Clomid or injectable?

A: In a word, no . . . but that doesn't mean they don't tell you something. Clomid often causes elevated BBTs around the time of taking the medication, and it appears to be more common to have a triphasic BBT on medications without pregnancy. It is also more common to have a long luteal phase without pregnancy. Other monitoring is more reliable when on medication.

Q: Will taking progesterone raise my BBTs?

A: It may raise your BBTs, but natural progesterone usually only causes a minor elevation (.1 or .2). Progestins like Provera can raise BBTs as well. Q: My BBTs were up for more than 18 days and I am not pregnant. Why?

A: That's a question for your doctor. If you were on medication for fertility problems, that could cause an extended luteal phase. It is also possible for a corpus luteal cyst to lead to a longer luteal phase. The best thing to do is see your doctor for a blood pregnancy test, exam and ultrasound.

Mucus Questions

Q: How can I tell fertile mucus from semen?

A: Fertile, egg-white mucus should stretch repeatedly in only one of two strands. Semen tends to be a little cloudier, and often stretches in several spider web-like strands. You may be able to stretch it a few times, but then it will begin to break.

Q: What is this about taking Robitussin to help with cervical mucus?

A: Plain Robitussin, or any generic with the guaifenesin as the only active ingredient, is an expectorant and helps thin mucus in your body, including cervical mucus. It does not create mucus for you, but can thin out thick mucus (a common side- effect of Clomid). The recommended dose is 2 teaspoons 3 times a day with a full glass of water, but you can take up to the maximum dose on the label. It should be started about 5 days before ovulation and continued through ovulation day. The water is very important since your body needs the fluid to create the mucus, and the guaifenesin can cause constipation. Being an herbalist, I prefer to use Yin-tonifying Chinese herbal formulas if indicated to address the root pattern.

Q: What are some sperm-friendly lubricants?

A: In our clinic, we most often recommend Preseed to use around ovulation. This lubricant is sperm-friendly and can a little goes a long way. Saliva is not a sperm- friendly medium, nor is water. Anything petroleum-based, such as Vaseline, should be avoided.

Chapter Three – The Infertility ABC's

Whether trying to understand your reproductive specialist's jargon or navigating endless fertility forums, the acronyms may be a bit confusing. Use this guide to prepare for your consult with your gynecologist or reproductive endocrinologist.

AH—Assisted hatching
The zona pellucida, or outer covering, of the embryo is partially opened, to aid implantation.

AMH- Anti-Mullerian hormone, measures ovarian reserve on a scale of 0-5.

ART—Assisted reproductive technology

A phrase to describe any treatments that involve handling human eggs or embryos.

CASA—Computer-assistedsemenanalysis
A laboratory technique to precisely measure and study sperm motion when male infertility is suspected.

CCCT—Clomiphene challenge test
A blood test to measure FSH (see below) taken on days three and 10 of the menstrual cycle. Clomiphene citrate is given on days five through nine to induce ovulation.

EEJ—Electro-ejaculation
A procedure that involves electrically stimulating tissue near a man's prostate to cause ejaculation.

FSH—Follicle stimulating hormone
A hormone produced by the pituitary gland (and sometimes given by injection). FSH stimulates the growth of the follicle surrounding an egg.

GIFT—Gamete intrafallopian transfer: The placing of sperm and egg directly into the fallopian tube, where fertilization takes place.

GnRH—Gonadotropin–releasing hormone
A hormone secreted by the hypothalamus (an area of the brain that controls reproduction and other actions) that prompts the pituitary gland to release FSH and LH into the bloodstream.

hCG—Human chorionic gonadotropin
A hormone produced by the placenta that is measured in common pregnancy tests. It may also be injected to stimulate ovulation and maturation of eggs.

HGH-Human Growth hormone
A hormone that increases the sensitivity of the ovaries to gonadotropin stimulation, and enhances follicular development

HMG—Human menopausal gonadotropin
A medication containing FSH and LH derived from the urine of postmenopausal women. HMG is used to stimulate the growth of multiple egg follicles.

HSG—Hysterosalpingogram
An X-ray procedure to determine whether the fallopian tubes are open to check for abnormalities in the uterus.

ICSI—Intracytoplasmic sperm injection
A procedure in which a single sperm is injected directly into an egg to help spur fertilization used primarily with male infertility.

IUI—Intrauterine insemination
A form of artificial insemination in which sperm that has been washed

free of seminal fluid to increase the chance of fertilization is inserted directly into the uterus.

IVF—In-vitro fertilization
A procedure in which an egg and sperm are combined in the laboratory to facilitate fertilization. Resulting embryos are transferred to a woman's uterus.

LH—Luteinizing hormone
Produced by the pituitary gland, this hormone normally causes a woman to ovulate and her eggs to mature.

OHSS—Ovarian hyperstimulation syndrome
A potentially life-threatening condition characterized by enlargement of the ovaries, fluid retention and weight gain that may occur when the ovaries are over-stimulated during assisted reproduction.

PESA—Percutaneous epididymal sperm aspiration
A procedure in which a needle is inserted into the gland that carries sperm from the testicle to the vas deferens in order to extract sperm for an IVF procedure.

PGD—Preimplantation genetic diagnosis
A test in which one or two cells are removed from an embryo and screened for genetic abnormalities.

TESE—Testicular sperm extraction
Surgery to remove testicular tissue and collect living sperm for use in an IVF or ICSI procedure.

Chapter Four: When to Seek Help

How long should I wait to seek help?

The general rule is if you are under 35 and have tried unsuccessfully to conceive for more than twelve months, then it might be a good time to at least get you and your partner evaluated. For women over 35 who have tried for more than six months without any luck, we often suggest that they check with their gynecologist to see if there is a need to seek specialized testing from an R.E.I. (reproductive endocrinologist and Infertility specialist). The beauty of working with techniques such as acupuncture and herbal medicine is that they are often diagnostic and therapeutic simultaneously. We often look for signs that the patient's hormones are becoming subtly more balanced in inquiring about improvement in sleep patterns, PMS symptoms, menstrual regularity and reduced clotting and pain, and overall mood. Our goal is to achieve this in three to six months, and to prepare our patient for a healthy pregnancy. If improvement in the above symptoms is not seen in this time frame, we are more likely to suspect a deeper issue and will then refer the patient directly to an REI.

A famous ancient Chinese medical text known as the Emperor's Book of Internal Medicine (Huang Di Nei Jing) written nearly 2,000 years ago describes the growth cycles of women in seven-year increments. The peak time of conception can be ascertained before the age of 35, which closely correlates to what a reproductive specialist advises their patients. Here are the seven cycles of seven listed in Nei Jing:

A woman's Kidney energy becomes prosperous at seven years of age (1x7). Her menstruation appears as the **ren** (sea of yin) channel flows

31

and the chong (sea of blood) channel becomes prosperous at the age of 14 (2x7).

Her Kidney qi reaches a balanced state, and her teeth are completely developed at the age of 21 (3x7).

Her vital energy and blood are substantial, her four limbs are strong and the body is at optimal condition at the age of 28 (4x7).
Her peak condition declines gradually. The yang ming channel is depleted, her face withers and her hair begins to fall out at the age of 35 (5x7).
Her three yang channels, tai yang, yang ming and shao yang, begin to decline. Her face complexion wanes and her hair turn white at the age of 42 (6x7).
The ren and chong channels are both declining, her menstruation ends, her physique turns old and feeble, and she can no longer conceive at the age of 49 (7x7).

Ironically, the cut off age for the majority of IVF clinics is around age 50 for those choosing donor egg cycles and 43 for those attempting IVF with their own eggs. During my hospital studies in China, I learned that women were commonly advised to marry at 20 and have a child by 25. If the couple did not fall pregnant by 26, the woman was often prescribed a Chinese herbal regimen to take for one year. If the couple had still not succeeded, other means such as acupuncture and IVF or medicated cycles were recommended. More and more, couples are delaying marriage and pregnancy until after their mid-thirties in the West and are then seeking treatment later than a typical Chinese couple would be. Therefore, Western acupuncture practitioners have combined herbal medicine and acupuncture along with integrated Western medicine in order to provide the best of both worlds.

Chapter Five: Overcoming Polycystic Ovarian Syndrome (PCOS)

April's Story:

I had my first menstrual cycle when I was 11 years old, and since then, have had very irregular cycles. I would have anywhere from 6 to 10 menstrual cycles a year, with no predictability whatsoever. I had painful and heavy periods as well. At times, I was doubled over in bed for a day or two with pain, as well as moodiness and irritability for a few days. When I hit my late teens, I began to develop a bad case of dark facial hair, and suffered with electrolysis and acne on my face that lasted for several years. I visited a few board-certified dermatologists and tried every prescription medication (other than Accutane), and the persistent acne would not resolve. I then tried other skin care specialists; many different types of skin care products and micro- dermabrasion and still could not get complete relief.

During my mid-twenties, I started researching my chronic medical conditions as a whole, and finally visited a renowned endocrinologist who diagnosed me with PCOS. Although I had already figured I had a hormonal imbalance, I was not happy with the diagnosis because I knew it might mean I would have a difficult time becoming pregnant. Both my endocrinologist and gynecologist suggested I take birth control pills to control the problem, and then switch to Metformin when I decide to try to conceive. I took birth control pills in my late teens and early twenties, and refused to ever take them again because I felt better off of them. I also read a lot about Metformin, and although women with PCOS were having success, I did not want to resort to medical intervention as a first resort without trying a more mild, natural approach. I researched various alternative therapies. At the same time as all of this was going on, I met my future husband and we got married in February of 2004. I was 30 years old.

I decided to try acupuncture, and happened upon Dr. Celada Duro's website. I gave her a call and scheduled my first treatment for June 24, 2004. At the same time, I charted my basal body temperature and took note of my cervical fluid. I diligently went for my weekly acupuncture appointments. Dr. Duro spent a lot of time with me during each appointment reviewing my current symptoms and asking me questions in order to tailor individualized treatment to meet my needs. She also mixed Chinese herbs every week in order to address my present symptoms. I diligently drank my herbs every day. At the same time, I was on absolutely no prescription medication or any other therapy. My cycles were still pretty long, and ranged anywhere from 40-50 days, but my premenstrual symptoms began to disappear. I did not feel as fatigued and foggy-brained during the day. I felt clearer and more energized. My husband noticed that I was barely moody and irritable when I got my periods. And, best of all, I never got one cystic pimple again! To this day, my skin remains clear and radiant. During my fourth cycle, and after about only 4 months of acupuncture, I got pregnant! My pregnancy was confirmed on December 15, 2004. I was ecstatic and felt great!

I continued acupuncture treatment during my entire first trimester, and am going back now for the last few weeks before labor. I have had an amazing and easy first pregnancy. I barely experienced any of the typical pregnancy symptoms that many women complain of, and have not missed a day of work due to the pregnancy. I am a true proponent of acupuncture therapy and Chinese herbs that are tailored for the individual in order to address fertility issues. The treatment is not time-consuming, and actually very relaxing. An entire course of acupuncture is also very reasonably priced, especially compared to conventional infertility treatment. I would also recommend acupuncture as an adjunct to conventional infertility treatment. I am 34 weeks pregnant and the happiest I have ever been in my life.

Despite the happy ending to her story, April was quite upset the first month she began using natural progesterone cream. Her BBT charts stretched into three pages, she rightly became concerned that this treatment was "screwing up her cycle" when her period did not appear. Happily, a pregnancy test confirmed what her temperatures were showing. Twenty days of a very high luteal phase translated into her first OBGYN visit that month! She proceeded beat the odds and have three more healthy beautiful children, naturally.

Polycystic ovarian syndrome (PCOS) is a common endocrine condition affecting millions of women worldwide. Women with PCOS may have enlarged ovaries that contain small collections of fluid — called follicles — located in each ovary as seen during an ultrasound exam and a host of other problems that go along with them, including anovulation (lack of ovulation) and menstrual abnormalities, hirsutism (facial hair), male pattern baldness, acne, and often obesity. Such women may also have varying degrees of insulin resistance and an increased incidence of Type II diabetes, unfavorable lipid patterns (usually high triglycerides), and a low bone density. Laboratory tests often show higher than normal circulating androgens, especially testosterone.

PCOS occurs when a woman doesn't ovulate, which causes a disruption in the normal, cyclical interrelationship among her hormones, brain and ovaries. Normally, the hypothalamus, a regulatory center in the brain, monitors the hormone output of the ovaries and synchronizes the normal menstrual cycle. When monthly bleeding ends, the hypothalamus secretes gonadotropin-releasing hormone (GnRH), which stimulates the pituitary gland in the brain to release follicle stimulating hormone (FSH) and luteinizing hormone (LH). These hormones direct an ovary to start making estrogen (mostly estradiol), and stimulate the maturation of eggs in multiple follicles.

As mentioned in women with PCOS, ovulation does not occur on a regular basis. Using hormone saliva testing for the past ten years in our clinic has revealed a pattern of estrogen dominance with progesterone

35

deficiency in the luteal phase. By supplementing the proper Chinese herbal medicine formula with normal physiologic doses of progesterone to treat PCOS, a normal menstrual cycle can return. If progesterone levels rise each month during the luteal phase of the cycle, as they are supposed to do, this maintains the normal synchronal pattern each month, and PCOS rarely, if ever, occurs. Natural progesterone should be the basis of PCOS treatment, along with attention to stress, exercise, and a diet low in refined sugars and carbohydrates.

If you have PCOS, you can use 15 to 20 mg of progesterone cream daily for the last two weeks of your cycle. The disappearance of facial hair and acne are usually obvious signs that hormones are becoming balanced, but to see these results, you'll need to give the treatment at least six months, in conjunction with proper diet and exercise. If your symptoms fade, try gradually easing off the progesterone (take half the dose, for example) and see how it goes. If your symptoms return, stay on the full dose for six more months.

Ideally, you would use the progesterone cream only during the months you need it, and encourage your body to return to its own normal hormonal rhythms as much as possible. It would also be helpful to check your hormone saliva levels from time to time by using a lab such as ZRT, testing during the luteal phase (around day 22 of your cycle). Some women with many damaged follicles may always need to supplement with a little bit of progesterone cream, and it can also work wonders for alleviating PMS.

Additionally, Chinese herbal medicine works to address subtle hormonal imbalances and can be instrumental in assisting the natural ebb and flow of your cycle. Ask your practitioner about a formula called Blossom, by Evergreen Herbs, to assist in creating a 28-30 day cycle. For some women with severe PCOS, they have never ovulated on their own and require prescription medication such as Provera or birth control to induce their cycles. Unfortunately, birth control is not the best plan when trying to conceive. However, even women who have never previously had a period on their own (or very infrequently) are thrilled to experience their first "real" cycle with the combination of herbal treatment and progesterone cream.

My Story

I remember like it was yesterday...the moment I decided to make a major change in the course of my life and pursue Chinese medicine studies. In the dark ages of the mid-to-late 1990's, before Google and Wikipedia, I was in undergraduate school and had no clue what was wrong with me. My cycles would come as go as they pleased, wreaking havoc on my hormones and sometimes disappearing for several months. No longer able to cope with what felt like weeks of never-ending PMS complete with bloating, mood swings and intolerable anxiety I decided to seek help. Four different gynecologists had all told me the same thing...that birth control was my only answer.

If only it had been so simple. As luck would have it, my body responds to birth control a like someone recovering from a hangover complete with nausea, headaches, chills and vomiting. Which brings me to the moment that changed my life. I was struck by a flying pack of birth control pills literally hurled at my head by my gynecologist and was told not to come back unless I'd taken the whole pack. I wasn't crazy...I was angry, and I knew there had to be a better approach.

That fateful checkup was nearly 20 years ago, but I still remember it so clearly because that day I made a promise to myself. I left that office in tears but I vowed to find an answer and to help other women when I did. At the age of 19, I left my premed studies and started acupuncture school. I discovered that what I was experiencing (undiagnosed PCOS) could be helped naturally and within six months I was having normal cycles for the first time in my life.

I have now been practicing Traditional Chinese Medicine for nearly half of my life and have devoted my practice to enhancing reproductive health naturally. My patients have been my greatest teachers and have inspired me to reach out to other women who might not have the support they need to do the previously unthinkable...take back control of their bodies without disguising their conditions with medications. Whether struggling with unexplained infertility, endometriosis, PCOS, or the devastating losses of repeated miscarriages, their desire to get to the root of the problem cannot be understated.

Here are the facts:

- **Hormonal imbalances from PCOS can lead to infertility, weight gain, acne, depression, and irregular cycles if left untreated**

- **Between five to 10 percent of women of childbearing age in the United States, or roughly 5 million, have PCOS and the number is climbing worldwide.**

- **Undiagnosed PCOS is extremely common, with over 50% of cases going unnoticed due to lack of education among providers and healthcare system in general**

- **The symptoms of PCOS can be reversed naturally, and the sooner they are addressed the better**

After nearly 20 years of working with PCOS in my own practice and kicking it to the curb personally, I felt compelled to offer more support for other women going through it. Just taking a supplement here and there or committing to an unsustainable diet is not the same as having a support system and tried-and-true plan in place. This program, aptly named the PCOS Revolution™ , has helped countless women overcome their struggles with PCOS though nutrition and supplement recommendations, exercise and the power of personalized group support.

PCOS doesn't have to be complicated, and in my experience I believe we can reverse the effects of PCOS by incorporating natural treatments such as proper diet, acupuncture, Chinese herbal medicine and natural progesterone. Although not an overnight process, it can be achieved with a little patience and diligence. Ideally, your team members should also include an understanding and experienced reproductive endocrinologist or gynecologist that will continue to monitor your glucose and hormone levels as your cycle stabilizes. An ultrasound every 6-12 months can also detect the health of your ovaries a signal a warning if your uterine lining has built up beyond healthy parameters.

In the following chapter, I have included a few recent research summaries of how acupuncture may work to support hormonal balance with PCOS. Please review these with your current acupuncturist to discuss what type of protocol could be most beneficial for you.

Chapter Five:
Acupuncture and PCOS

Current evidence of acupuncture on polycystic ovarian syndrome

Lim CE, Wong WS. Gynecol Endocrinol. 2010 Mar 16. [Epub ahead of print]
Faculty of Medicine, South Western Sydney Clinical School, University of New South Wales, Sydney, Australia.

Objective. This paper aims to provide a literature review on evaluating the efficacy of acupuncture therapy in the treatment of polycystic ovarian syndrome (PCOS) by reviewing clinical trials; randomized and non-randomized and observational studies on PCOS. The paper will also determine the possible mechanism of acupuncture treatment in PCOS, limitations of recruited studies and suggest further improvements in future studies. Design. A comprehensive literature search was conducted through the databases Medline, PubMed, EMBASE, Cochrane, AMED (Allied and Complementary Medicine), NCCAM (The National Centre for Complementary and Alternative Medicine) to identify relevant monographs. Results. Four studies were recruited. Several studies showed that acupuncture significantly increases beta-endorphin levels for periods up to 24 h and may have regulatory effect on FSH, LH and androgen. beta-endorphin increased levels secondary to acupuncture affects the hyperthalamic-pituitary-adrenal (HPA) axis through promoting the release of ACTH through stimulation of its precursor pro-opiomelanocortinsynthesis. Inclusion criteria: All available acupuncture studies on human subjects with PCOS from June 1970 to June 2009. Exclusion criteria: Studies not meeting the inclusion criteria, published in languages other than English or animal studies.

Conclusion: **Acupuncture is a safe and effective treatment to PCOS as the adverse effects of pharmacologic interventions are not expected by women with PCOS**. Acupuncture therapy may have a role in PCOS by: increasing of blood flow to the ovaries, reducing of ovarian volume and the number of ovarian cysts, controlling hyperglycemia through increasing insulin sensitivity and decreasing blood glucose and insulin levels, reducing cortisol levels and assisting in weight loss and anorexia. However, well-designed, randomized controlled trials are needed to elucidate the true effect of acupuncture on PCOS.

Effect of electro acupuncture combined with auricular point tapping and pressing on serum insulin and testosterone in the patients of obese women with polycystic ovary syndrome

Xu J, Qu HQ, Fang HLXu J, Qu HQ, Fang HLZhongguo Zhen Jiu. 2009 Jun;29(6):441-3.

OBJECTIVE: To assess the therapeutic effect and mechanism of electro acupuncture combined with auricular point tapping and pressing on the obese women with polycystic ovary syndrome. METHODS: Thirty-nine cases of obese women with polycystic ovary syndrome were treated with electro- acupuncture combined with auricular point tapping and pressing, body points as Tianshu (ST 25), Fenglong (ST 40), Guanyuan (CV 4) and Siman (KI 14) etc. were selected, and ear points as Kou (mouth), Wei (stomach) and Pi (spleen) etc. were selected. After 3 courses, the therapeutic effect, the body mass index (BMI), the waist circumference (WC) and the changes of the serum insulin (Ins) and testosterone (T) were compared before and after treatment. RESULTS: Of the 39 cases, 10 cases were cured, 25 cases were effective, 4 cases were ineffective, with a total effective rate of 89.7%; there were significant differences in BMI, WC, Ins and T of the patients compared with that before treatment (all P < 0.01).

CONCLUSION: **Electroacupuncture combined with auricular point tapping and pressing has a good clinical effect on obese women with polycystic ovary syndrome, the treatment mechanism may realized by regulating the serum.**

Low-frequency electro acupuncture and physical exercise decrease high muscle sympathetic nerve activity in polycystic ovary syndrome.

Stener-Victorin E, Jedel E, Janson PO, Sverrisdottir YB. Institute of Neuroscience and Physiology, Dept. of Physiology, Sahlgrenska Academy, Univ. of Gothenburg, Box 434, SE-405 30 Göteborg, Sweden. elisabet.stener-victorin@neuro.gu.se Am J Physiol Regul Integr Comp Physiol. 2009 Aug;297(2): R387-95. Epub 2009 Jun 3.

We have recently shown that polycystic ovary syndrome (PCOS) is associated with high muscle sympathetic nerve activity (MSNA). Animal studies support the concept that low-frequency electro acupuncture (EA) and physical exercise, via stimulation of ergoreceptors and somatic afferents in the muscles, may modulate the activity of the sympathetic nervous system. The aim of the present study was to investigate the effect of these interventions on sympathetic nerve activity in women with PCOS. In a randomized controlled trial, 20 women with PCOS were randomly allocated to one of three groups: low-frequency EA (n = 9), physical exercise (n = 5), or untreated control (n = 6) during 16 wk. Direct recordings of multiunit efferent postganglionic MSNA in a muscle fascicle of the peroneal nerve before and following 16 wk of treatment. Biometric, hemodynamic, endocrine, and metabolic parameters were measured. Low-frequency EA (P = 0.036) and physical exercise (P = 0.030) decreased MSNA burst frequency compared with the untreated control group. The low-frequency EA group reduced sagittal diameter (P = 0.001), while the physical exercise group reduced body weight (P = 0.004) and body mass index (P = 0.004) compared with the untreated control group. Sagittal diameter was related to MSNA burst frequency (Rs = 0.58, P < 0.005) in the EA group. No correlation was found for body mass index and MSNA in the exercise group. There were no differences between the groups in hemodynamic, endocrine, and metabolic variables. **For the first time we demonstrate that low-frequency EA and physical exercise lowers high sympathetic nerve activity in women with PCOS. Thus treatment with low-frequency EA or physical exercise with the aim to reduce MSNA may be of importance for women with PCOS.**

Acupuncture and PCOS anovulation: Electro-Acupuncture induces regular ovulations Effects of electro-acupuncture on anovulation in women with polycystic ovary syndrome.

Stener-Victorin E, Waldenstrom U,Tagnfors U, Lundeberg T, Lindstedt G, Janson PO. Department of Obstetrics and Gynecology, Goteborg University, Sweden.

BACKGROUND: The present study was designed to evaluate if electro-acupuncture (EA) could affect oligo-/anovulation and related endocrine and neuro-endocrine parameters in women with polycystic ovary syndrome (PCOS). METHODS: Twenty-four women (between the ages of 24 and 40 years) with PCOS and oligo-/amenorrhea were included in this non-randomized, longitudinal, prospective study. The study period was defined as the period extending from 3 months before the first EA treatment, to 3 months after the last EA treatment (10-14 treatments), in total 8-9 months. The menstrual and ovulation patterns were confirmed by recording of vaginal bleedings and by daily registrations of the basal body temperature (BBT). Blood samples were collected within a week before the first EA, within a week after the last EA and 3 months after EA. RESULTS: Nine women (38%) experienced a good effect. They displayed a mean of 0.66 ovulations/woman and month in the period during and after the EA period compared to a mean of 0.15 before the EA period (p=0.004). Before EA, women with a good effect had a significantly lower body-mass index (BMI) (p<0.001), waist-to-hip circumference ratio (WHR) (p=0.0058), serum testosterone concentration (p=0.0098), serum testosterone/sex hormone binding globulin (SHBG) ratio (p=0.011) and serum basal insulin concentration (p=0.0054), and a significantly higher concentration of serum SHBG (p=0.040) than did those women with no effect.

CONCLUSION: **Repeated EA treatments induce regular ovulations in more than one third of the women with PCOS. The group of women with good effect had a less androgenic hormonal profile before treatment and a less pronounced metabolic disturbance compared with the group with no effect. For this selected group EA offers an alternative to pharmacological ovulation induction.**

Hypothalamic neuroendocrine functions in rats with dihydrotestosterone-induced polycystic ovary syndrome: effects of low-frequency electro-acupuncture.

Feng Y, Johansson J, Shao R, Mannerås L, Fernandez-Rodriguez J, Billig H, Stener-Victorin E. Institute of Neuroscience and Physiology, Department of Physiology, Sahlgrenska Academy, UniversityofGothenburg,Gothenburg,SwedenPLoS ONE4(8):e6638.doi:10.1371/journal.pone.000663848

Adult female rats continuously exposed to androgens from prepuberty have reproductive and metabolic features of polycystic ovary syndrome (PCOS). We investigated whether such exposure adversely affects estrous cyclicity and the expression and distribution of gonadotropin-releasing hormone (GnRH), GnRH receptors, and corticotrophin-releasing hormone (CRH) in the hypothalamus and whether the effects are mediated by the androgen receptor (AR). We also assessed the effect of low-frequency electro-acupuncture (EA) on those variables. At 21 days of age, rats were randomly divided into three groups (control, PCOS, and PCOS EA; n = 12/group) and implanted subcutaneously with 90-day continuous-release pellets containing vehicle or 5alpha- dihydrostestosterone (DHT). From age 70 days, PCOS EA rats received 2-Hz EA (evoking muscle twitches) five times/week for 4-5 weeks. Hypothalamic protein expression was measured by immunohistochemistry and western blot. DHT-treated rats were acyclic, but controls had regular estrous cycles. In PCOS rats, hypothalamic medial preoptic AR protein expression and the number of AR- and GnRH-immunoreactive cells were increased, but CRH was not affected; however, GnRH receptor expression was decreased in both the pituitary and hypothalamus. Low- frequency EA restored estrous cyclicity within 1 week and reduced the elevated hypothalamic GnRH and AR expression levels. EA did not affect GnRH receptor or CRH expression. Interestingly, nuclear AR co-localized with GnRH in the hypothalamus. Thus, rats with DHT-induced PCOS have disrupted estrous cyclicity and an increased number of hypothalamic cells expressing GnRH, most likely mediated by AR activation. **Repeated low-frequency EA normalized estrous cyclicity and restored GnRH and AR protein expression. These results may help explain the beneficial neuroendocrine effects of low-frequency EA in women with PCOS.**

Acupuncture and exercise restore adipose tissue expression of sympathetic markers and improve ovarian morphology in rats with dihydrotestosterone-induced PCOS

Manneras L. Cajander S. Lonn M. Stener-Victorin E.

Department of Physiology, Sahlgrenska Academy, University of Gothenburg, Gothenburg, Sweden. American Journal of Physiology - Regulatory Integrative and Comparative Physiology. 2009; 296(4)(pp R1124-R1131),

Altered activity of the sympathetic nervous system, which innervates adipose and ovarian tissue, may play a role in polycystic ovary syndrome (PCOS). We hypothesize that electro-acupuncture (EA) and physical exercise reduce sympathetic activity by stimulating ergoreceptors and somatic afferent pathways in muscles. Here we investigated the effects of low-frequency EA and physical exercise on mRNA expression of sympathetic markers in adipose tissue and on ovarian morphology in female rats that received dihydrotestosterone (DHT) continuously, starting before puberty, to induce PCOS. At age 11 wk, rats with DHT-induced PCOS were randomly divided into three groups: PCOS, PCOS plus EA, and PCOS plus exercise. The latter two groups received 2-Hz EA (evoking muscle twitches) three times/week or had free access to a running wheel for 4-5 wk. In mesenteric adipose tissue, expression of beta3-adrenergic receptor (ADRB3), nerve growth factor (NGF), and neuropeptide Y (NPY) mRNA was higher in untreated PCOS rats than in controls. Low-frequency EA and exercise down regulated mRNA expression of NGF and NPY, and EA also down regulated expression of ADRB3, compared with untreated rats with DHT-induced PCOS. EA and exercise improved ovarian morphology, as reflected in a higher proportion of healthy antral follicles and a thinner theca interna cell layer than in untreated PCOS rats. **These findings support the theory that increased sympathetic activity contributes to the development and maintenance of PCOS and that the effects of EA and exercise may be mediated by modulation of sympathetic outflow to the adipose tissue and ovaries.**

Effects of electro acupuncture on in vitro fertilization and embryo transplantation in the patient of infertility with different syndromes

[Article in Chinese] Cui W, Liu LL, Sun W, Kong W. Second Affiliated Hospital of Shandong University of TCM, Jinan, China. cuiwei9996@sohu.com
Zhongguo Zhen Jiu. 2008 Apr; 28(4): 254-6.

OBJECTIVE: To probe into effects of electro acupuncture (EA) on in vitro fertilization and embryo transplantation (IVF-ET) in the patient of infertility with different syndromes. METHODS: Among the 126 patients of infertility who received EA for IVF-ET, 52 cases of kidney deficiency type (group A), 44 cases of the liver-qi stag- nation type (group B) and 30 cases of phlegm- dampness type (group C) were selected. All of them in the 3 groups were treated with EA before and during con- trolled ovarian hyper-stimulation, and the effects of EA on the patients in the 3 groups were investigated.

RESULTS: The fertility rate, implantation rate and clinical pregnancy rate were 81.3%, 23.5%, 44.1% in group A, 80.5%, 27.8%, 46.5% in group B and 71.9%, 17.1%, 32.7% in group C, respectively, group A and B being better than group C ($P<0.05$) ; the good quality embryo rate of 70.7% in group B was significantly higher than 57.9% in group C ($P<0.05$); there were no significant differences in patient's basal condition, the dosage and administration time of gonadotropin, and blood level of estradiol on the day of injection of human chorionic gonadotropin, the number of gained oocytes, oocyte cleavage rate and the number of transplantation embryo among the 3 groups.

CONCLUSION: **Clinical effects of EA treatment on IVF-ET in the infertility patients of kidney deficiency type and the patients of the liver-qi stagnation type are better than that in the patients of phlegm-dampness type.**

Acupuncture in assisted reproductive technology and PCOS.

Stener-Victorin E. Von Hagens C. Gynakologische Endokrinologie.
6(2)(pp 67-71), 2008
Department of Physiology/Endocrinology, Sahlgrenska Academy,
Goteborg University, Goteborg, Sweden.

In controlled trials, acupuncture alleviated pain during oocyte
aspiration for in vitro fertilization/embryo transfer (IVF/ET) treatment
and regulated uterine and ovarian blood flow. Recent clinical and
experimental data on the effect of acupuncture in polycystic ovary
syndrome (PCOS) clearly demonstrate that acupuncture affects PCOS
via modulation of endocrine, neuroendocrine and endogenous
regulatory systems and exerts long-lasting beneficial effects on
ovulation and on metabolic and endocrine systems. Some trials even
suggest that acupuncture at embryo transfer has a positive impact on
pregnancy rates. Results of recent trials are discussed, as are the
difficulties and confounders associated with the interpretation of
controlled trials and an attempt to standardize reporting of acupuncture
interventions (STRICTA). **Acupuncture is a safe intervention in the
hands of competent practitioners and is low in cost, but well-
designed studies are lacking. Clinicians and scientists are
encouraged to conduct large, prospective, randomized trials to
demonstrate more precisely the physiological impact of
acupuncture on the reproductive system and its possible impact on
pregnancy rates.**

**Acupuncture in polycystic ovary syndrome: Current experimental
and clinical evidence.**

Stener-Victorin E.Jedel E. Manneras L Institute of Neuroscience and
Physiology, Department of Physiology, Goteborg University,

Goteborg, Sweden. Journal of Neuroendocrinology. 20(3)(pp. 290-298), 2008

This review describes the aetiology and pathogenesis of polycystic ovary syndrome (PCOS) and evaluates the use of acupuncture to prevent and reduce symptoms related with PCOS. PCOS is the most common female endocrine disorder and it is strongly associated with hyperandrogenism, ovulatory dysfunction and obesity. PCOS increases the risk for metabolic disturbances such as hyperinsulinemia and insulin resistance, which can lead to type 2 diabetes, hypertension and an increased likelihood of developing cardiovascular risk factors and impaired mental health later in life. Despite extensive research, little is known about the aetiology of PCOS. The syndrome is associated with peripheral and central factors that influence sympathetic nerve activity. Thus, the sympathetic nervous system may be an important factor in the development and maintenance of PCOS. Many women with PCOS require prolonged treatment. Current pharmacological approaches are effective but have adverse effects. Therefore, nonpharmacological treatment strategies need to be evaluated. Clearly, acupuncture can affect PCOS via modulation of endogenous regulatory systems, including the sympathetic nervous system, the endocrine and the neuroendocrine system. **Experimental observations in rat models of steroid-induced polycystic ovaries and clinical data from studies in women with PCOS suggest that acupuncture exerts long-lasting beneficial effects on metabolic and endocrine systems and ovulation.**

Clinical study on needle-pricking therapy for treatment of polycystic ovarian syndrome

Chen D. Chen SR. Shi XL. Guo FL. Zhu YK. Li S. Cai MX. Deng LH. Xu H. Zhongguo Zhenjiu. 27(2):99-102, 2007 Feb. The First Affiliated

Hospital of Jinan University, Guangzhou 510630, China.
drchendong@yahoo.com.cn[Chinese]

OBJECTIVE: To probe into the clinical effect of needle-pricking therapy for treatment of polycystic ovarian syndrome. METHODS: One hundred and twenty-one cases of polycystic ovarian syndrome were divided into a needle-pricking therapy group of 61 cases and a medication group of 60 cases with randomized and controlled method. The needle-pricking therapy group were treated by needle-pricking therapy at sacral plexus stimulating points on both sides of the spine and lateral points of Dazhui (CV 14), and the medication group by oral administration of Clomiphene and intramuscular injection of chorionic gonadotropin (HCG). Levels of hormones and symptoms in the patients before treatment, after treatment of 3 cycles and at the sixth cycle after treatment were investigated.

RESULTS: After treatment of 3 cycles, the level of hormone and B type ultrasound examination were significantly improved in the two groups ($P < 0.01$). At the sixth cycle after treatment, the conditions of the patients in the medication group were returned to the original levels before treatment, while the conditions in the needle-pricking therapy group still kept at the post-therapeutic level, and their menstruation and ovulation restored to normal state, and the ovulation mucosa and the pregnancy rate were significantly higher than those in the medication group (all $P < 0.01$).

CONCLUSION: **Needle-pricking therapy has obvious effect on polycystic ovarian syndrome, and has a good long-term therapeutic effect.**

Application of acupuncture in intrauterine insemination in patients with polycystic ovary syndrome.

Wang W.-J. Gao T.-Department of Rehabilitation Medicine, Guangdong Second People's Hospital, Guangzhou 510317 Guangdong Province, China.
Journal of Clinical Rehabilitative Tissue Engineering Research.11(39)(pp.7996- 7998),2007.

Aim: To summarize the influence of acupuncture on intrauterine insemination (IUI) in patients with polycystic ovary syndrome (PCOS) and its application through the study of recent ten-year relevant literatures. Methods: The articles of influence of acupuncture on patients with PCOS were searched for in China Journal Full-text Database (CJFD) published from January 1996 to June 2006 with the key words of "acupuncture, polycystic ovary syndrome, intrauterine insemination" in Chinese. At the same time, Elsevier-SDOL database was undertaken to identify the relevant articles published between January 1996 and June 2006 with the same key words in English. Results: The selected articles should be as follows: the effect of acupuncture on PCOS patients, the application of acupuncture to IUI, the influential factors during IUI and study of acupuncture on this aspect. Totally 200 articles of the effect of acupuncture on PCOS patients, 300 of the influential factors during IUI, 30 of the application of acupuncture to IUI were collected, and 16 of them were accorded with the criteria. Most former study had focused on acupuncture for PCOS and clinical research of acupuncture for improving ovulation. It thought that acupuncture could effectively cure PCOS, improve ovulation by stimulating ovary, and believed that acupuncture for improving ovulation not only had no side effect, but also could get good curative effect, which was stable and unvarying. Besides, German scholars found that if acupuncture therapy was used in insemination externalis or intracytoplasmic sperm injection (ICSI), the successful rate of pregnancy was nearly 50%. However, there was no report of the application of acupuncture to IUI in patients with PCOS at abroad.

Conclusion: **IUI has been widely used in the treatment of infertility, and acupuncture has better accelerated effect on ovulation. Therefore, acupuncture therapy can be applied before and after IUI in PCOS patients so as to study the application of acupuncture that induces ovulation to IUI in PCOS patients and observe the successful rate of IUI in PCOS patients due to acupuncture.**

Chapter Six: Male Factor Infertility

Throughout the process of fertility treatment, it can seem like it's "all about the female," yet nearly half of the causes of infertility have been attributed to male factor issues in recent years. Much of the reasoning for sweeping men under the rug has been due to the advent of ICSI (intracytoplasmic sperm injection) during IVF, which only requires one healthy sperm per egg. The advice of practitioners of Chinese medicine has been to address the couple holistically, and achieve the best state of health for both prior to embarking on a round of ART (assisted reproductive techniques).

Why Are Men Infertile?

Recent statistics show that abnormal semen parameters can be identified in up to 50% of infertile couples. Most commonly, the cause is unknown. The role of oxidative stress has proven to be an integral part of male subfertility. Causes of oxidative stress include infection, industrial compounds, cigarette smoking and tobacco use, elevated temperatures, strenuous exercise, and trauma. The most widely studied type of oxidant is known as reactive oxygen species (ROS), which may be found in white blood cells and produced by sperm.

When the balance of the body's ability to balance antioxidant production against ROS occurs, the sperm's ability to repair or compensate for damage is overwhelmed. This can result in DNA damage, decreased motility and compromised sperm membrane integrity. Antioxidants act to protect against oxidative stress and damage, sort of like a cleanup crew after a rock concert. These antioxidants are present within sperm and seminal plasma and can be improved by incorporating certain dietary suggestions. Adversely, lower intake of antioxidants can be associated with poor semen quality.

When I meet with a couple for the first time, I find that the female partner has often had her fallopian tubes and hormone levels checked by her gynecologist, but the male partner has yet to have a semen analysis. In the course of the consultation, I sometimes will discuss the case of a couple in their late twenties who had been trying to conceive on their own for five years. The wife had undergone the appropriate testing by her OBGYN and was diagnosed with PCOS. She had been prescribed Clomid for several months to no avail when they decided to try acupuncture and found our office.

On the initial intake, I saw that the husband had undergone an inguinal hernia repair at age 5, but no further surgeries were listed. At my urging, he underwent a semen analysis that concluded there were no healthy sperm to be found-a heart-breaking diagnosis of azoospermia. The couple was shocked and saddened that so much time had been wasted and immediately went for a consultation at a local IVF clinic where they were treated in conjunction with acupuncture. The cost of the semen analysis was $200. The time that they saved by changing their plan from natural treatment to IVF was priceless.

Not all cases are this severe, but men if there's one thing that you can do to appease your partner, it would be to volunteer a semen sample when you see there might be trouble on the fertility horizon. Even in the event where the analysis comes back slightly abnormal or low, there are multitudes of ways to improve your sperm quality within 2-3 months of treatment. And if your results come back normal or above average, that's just one less problem you have to worry about.

Suggestions For Improving Male Factor Infertility:

-Vitamin C 500 mg per day (Protects against and improves DNA damage, improves motility and concentration). Use 1000 mg per day for agglutination issues.

-L-Carnitine 500 mg per day (improves concentration, motility, and morphology, along with total oxidative capacity)

-Co-enzyme Q10 200 mg per day (improves motility and concentration, along with fertilization with ICSI for men treated with 60mg/day for 3.5 months)

In addition to this protocol, we recommend acupuncture treatment once weekly for 12 weeks, then refer for a follow up semen analysis for comparison. In moderate-to-borderline oligospermia, we see an average of 30-40% improvement in all parameters. Since sperm are regenerated every 70-90 days, this provides a wonderful opportunity to measure results and repeat the protocol if necessary. Whether contemplating a medicated cycle or trying naturally, it is extremely important to treat both partners with acupuncture and supplements to provide the healthiest outcome for pregnancy. After all, there is never any harm in having too many healthy sperm!

Male Health According to the Huang Di Nei Jing, circa 200 A.D.: Male Jing Cycles of Eight

A man's Kidney energy is prosperous, his hair develops and his teeth emerge at the age of eight (1x 8).
His Kidney energy grows and is filled with vital energy, and he is able to let his sperm out at the age of 16 (2x8).
His Kidney energy is developed, his extremities are strong, and all of his teeth are developed by the age of 24 (3x8).
His body has developed to its best condition, and his extremities and muscles are very strong at the age of 32 (4x8).
His Kidney energy begins to decline, his hair falls out and his teeth begin to whither at the age of 40 (5x8).

His Kidney energy declines more, the yang energy of the entire body declines, his complexion becomes withered and his hair turns white at the age of 48 (6x8). His Liver energy declines as a result of Kidney deficiency; the tendons become rigid and fail to be nimble at the age of 56 (7x8).

His essence and vital energy is weak, as are his bones and tendons. His teeth fall out and his body becomes decrepit at the age of 64 (8x8).

As research yields new evidence of how we can turn back the clock on our reproductive system, both partners can benefit from adopting healthier lifestyles and at minimum, reducing stress that can seem so inherent to the infertility treatment process.

Chapter Seven: Choosing The Right Treatment: Natural, Medicated or Both

In addition to worrying about your "ticking clock," you must also seek out the right specialists who will provide the tools you need to be successful on your journey. Throughout the years, we have found that a combination approach of compassion, science, and trust provide the best treatment outcome. Only focusing on your ovaries might get you through the first round of IVF or IUI, but what if that's not successful? How do you have the strength emotionally to endure another cycle, or to subject your body to another round of hormones?

Research into the causes of drop out rates at IVF centers found that the decision was mostly due to the fact that the couple was spent emotionally rather than financially. The financial burden of spending thousands of dollars on an IVF treatment that may end in a negative pregnancy test or miscarriage cannot be underestimated and may contribute to the disintegration of an already- strained marriage.

By integrating different approaches such as counseling, acupuncture, mind-body groups and nutrition, the odds of conception can be increased. Acupuncture has been proven to lower the effects of stress inherent in IVF treatment. The positive effects are improved outlook on the treatment plan and better "frame of min d" going into the transfer. For further research on combining acupuncture with IVF and treatment outcomes, see chapter 14 at the end of this book.

Whether you go the strictly traditional route, purely holistic, or a combination of both will depend on a multitude of factor s. The general rule with infertility is the more complicated the picture, the longer the treatment time. By having an understanding of you and your partner's optimal timeline, you may set a "fertility deadline" by opting to try naturally for six months to one year, then moving to a medicated cycle of Clomid or IUI if you are still not pregnant. That said, a couple in their forties may be on a completely different timeline than their thirty-something year- old friends. If you are planning to travel for extending periods or foresee a particularly stressful period of your life coming up, it may be wise to delay medicated treatment until your stress level is more manageable.

The Second Opinion

During the course of fertility treatment, navigating through the maze of information on when to schedule which procedure or test can be frightening. If you have been under the care of a knowledgeable, compassionate reproductive specialist who has walked you through the initial testing and created a solid care plan for you, congratulations on finding the right one! In reality, you might be wondering if it's time to seek another opinion if you have any lingering doubts that some stones have been unturned. At our office, we work with several reproductive endocrinologists that integrate acupuncture and proven supplements into their treatment plan.

Evaluating Your Fertility

Have you been on the same fertility treatment protocol for 3 cycles or more?

Yes: Most fertility doctors will advise that if you haven't seen success in 3 cycles, it's time to move on. Try working with your doctor to tweak your medication levels or incorporate acupuncture into your treatment plan.

No: It can take up to 3 cycles to see success with a particular fertility treatment, but don't waste time on a treatment that isn't working for you. Time is of the essence when it comes to fertility!

Have you been sticking to a specific fertility treatment for financial reasons?

Yes: Try reviewing your infertility insurance coverage one more time. Make sure you are clear on what fertility treatments, diagnostics, or surgical procedures for fertility are covered and what's not. It doesn't hurt to call the insurance company, either. If you don't have coverage or you only have coverage for some less invasive treatments, call your fertility clinic's financial advisor. This person will have an idea of what your insurance covers and will talk to you about financing options at your clinic. You can also look into outside financing options. In some cases, moving to a higher-tech treatment like IVF can be less expensive in the long run versus multiple IUI cycles.

No: If finances aren't the reason you've been hung up on a particular fertility treatment, ask yourself what is the reason. Is it fear of the unknown? Comfort? Feeling like you're only a number and not a person? Remember, the goal of fertility treatment is to get you the baby you've been longing for. You shouldn't do anything that is against your personal morals, but sometimes a fresh start is exactly what you need.

Do you understand your fertility doctor's plans for your upcoming cycle?

Yes: Good. It is important to advocate for your own health, especially when it comes to making a baby. Don't be afraid to ask questions and make phone calls. No one else will do these things for you. .

No: Call your fertility doctor and ask for clarification. In many cases, your doctor wants you to be a part of the fertility treatment team. They will help you to understand the protocol and you should voice your concerns, if any. If your doctor isn't available to answer your questions before your next cycle, ask your fertility nurse. They are there to help.

Is your doctor comfortable with your your suggestions of complementary medicine in conjunction with your treatment plan?

Yes: You've learned that no one knows more about your body than you and found the right team to take you to the next step. Your doctor (or nurse) is prepared to answer any concerns or questions you may have about the use of supplements and/or acupuncture prior to and during your IVF/IUI cycle and you feel at ease with them.

No: Consider writing down your questions before your next visit and determine whether your doctor will be open to reviewing your situation on an individual basis. Your fertility center might not have acupuncture on-site on the day of embryo transfer, for example, but they may provide you with recommendations of fertility acupuncturists in the area. Make sure you communicate with your acupuncturist your doctor's wishes if they have recommended against the use of certain supplements.

Do you feel uneasy about one aspect of your treatment, but are afraid to speak up?

Yes: If something doesn't sound right to you, question it. Be the squeaky wheel! Your doctor will explain why they have chosen a specific fertility treatment protocol. If you're still not satisfied after getting clarification, it may be time for a second opinion.

No: Sounds like you're one of the fertility treatment team. Great job! If at any time you do feel leery about the fertility treatment plan, speak up. It's the best thing you can do for yourself and your future baby!

Have you been considering a second opinion, but you just haven't taken the leap yet?

Yes: Surprisingly, fertility patients report the reason they haven't sought out a second opinion as fear of insulting their fertility doctor. The truth is, your doctor knows just as well as you do that a good fit is important. If you aren't getting a good vibe, remember this is a professional relationship and your care is dependent upon it. Don't look at it as "breaking up" with your fertility doctor- they have your best interests in mind and often take your feedback to improve their practice. It is a step in the right direction for treating your fertility.

No: Should you consider a second opinion? Take all of the above factors into consideration to ensure you are comfortable with your fertility treatment. Start this year fresh and confident that you WILL reach your goal of having a baby!

Chapter Eight: Asking For Medical Records

At our clinic, we often ask patients to bring their medical records with them so that we can better understand the extent of their infertility diagnosis. It is your right as a patient to obtain your medical records from your doctor but I find most patients have no record of past hormone level testing, surgical history or even basic physical exam checkups. I am including a checklist of common tests that should be or might have already been performed as part of a fertility workup. They will differ according to what IVF clinic you visit, but it is a good outline of what is recommended by the majority of them.

Fill in the chart as you would a vaccine record, with date and result of test performed. Since most IVF clinics like to see that you've had an HSG (hysterosalpingogram) within the last 12 months prior to embarking on an IVF cycle, it's a good thing to know if your gynecologist might have performed one and what the results were.

Once the tests are performed, ask for a copy of your results. Some clinics charge a small fee for copying and mailing your records, so make sure to ask beforehand. If you are requesting records from your current doctor, specify that you are not jumping ship but want to have a completed file for your records. The general rule at most IVF centers is that prior labs and imaging needs to be performed within a year of the start of your medicated cycle in order to not be repeated again.

Owning a copy of your medical records can save both time and money by avoiding the repetition of testing and will be appreciated by other members of your fertility healthcare team. Besides, you paid for it, right?

Possible Medical Tests-Female

- Hormone levels (FSH, LH, E2, prolactin, DHEA, mid-luteal serum progesterone)

- Thyroid Panel

- HSG (Hysterosalpingography)

- General physical exam and PAP

- Pelvic Ultrasound, Laparoscopy, Hysteroscopy, or SIS

- Laparoscopic surgery D&C

- LEEP

- Myomectomy Endometrial biopsy

- Genetic tests (both partners) Miscarriage Panel and/or Autoimmune Testing

Possible Medical Tests-Male

- Basic or Complex Semen Analysis General physical exam

- Hormone testing (including thyroid panel)

- Scrotal Ultrasound

*Please note that the above tests are not comprehensive and are not recommended for everyone. Which testing you have performed is largely up to your doctor's discretion.

Results and Date Performed-Female:

Results and Date Performed-Male:

Other testing and notes:

Chapter Nine: Acupuncture and Herbal Medicine for Infertility

What do Mariah Carey and Celine Dion have in common? Besides their superstar celebrity status, both used acupuncture to get pregnant. As media coverage of acupuncture's role in the treatment of infertility increases, certain questions repeatedly arise from prospective patients. As an acupuncturist specializing in infertility, I will attempt to clarify as much as possible the benefits and drawbacks to beginning a course of acupuncture and Chinese herbal medicinal treatment.

What is Oriental Medicine and how does it help with infertility?

Oriental Medicine has developed over thousands of years to include acupuncture, Chinese herbal medicine, tui-na (soft tissue mobilization), and qigong (meditative breathing and movement). The most popular branch of Oriental Medicine in the West, however, is acupuncture. Acupuncture has been proven to increase success rates of IVF by nearly twenty percent when administered in a German study in 2004. Of course, Chinese doctors have known of the benefits of Oriental Medicine in the treatment of infertility long before it was ever studied in the West, with the first known publications on infertility appearing several hundred years ago. Due to recent studies, we now know that acupuncture affects the pituitary gland and acts on the sympathetic nervous system to reduce stress and regulate hormones. In the treatment of infertility, it has also been shown to increase blood flow to the uterus. Herbal medicine has been rigorously studied in China and some herbs have been shown to increase sperm motility in men and balance estrogen and progesterone in women.

Both of my fallopian tubes are blocked, can acupuncture help?

In this case, ART (assisted reproduction technology), rather than acupuncture, would be recommended. Unfortunately, some patients in this situation pursue "natural" therapies too long when their main or only choice of success is IVF.

What types of infertility respond best to Oriental Medicine?

Relatively minor complications such as slightly low sperm counts, irregular ovulation, mild endometriosis, and vague hormonal imbalances tend to respond the fastest. More severe cases of anovulation and moderate to severe endometriosis can be improved but can take longer than the usual three months of treatment. Acupuncture and Chinese herbal medicine often can correct such imbalances successfully in younger women. Those with infertility due to PCOS also fit into this category. Women over forty might do better with a combination of ART and Oriental Medicine.

My doctor doesn't want me to take herbs during my IVF cycle; will the acupuncture alone be effective?

While no treatment is 100% guaranteed, acupuncture without Chinese herbs can still be quite effective. Many IVF clinics ask their patients to avoid herbs during a stimulated cycle, which is good advice considering the strong medications that are circulating in the patient's body. However, in a case where a woman is over the age of 40 and has undergone several unsuccessful IVF and ART attempts already, Chinese medicine might be recommended along with acupuncture (with the agreement of the patient's doctor) to increase her chances of pregnancy.

Should my partner be undergoing acupuncture and herbal treatment as well?

In Oriental medicine theory, both partners should address their health in order to achieve the best outcome. As it takes nearly 90 days for sperm to develop, men are usually asked to begin treatment as early as possible in the case of mildly low sperm count. Additionally, nutritional recommendations are made to maximize treatment benefits. Acupuncture can also assist both partners by decreasing stress and promoting relaxation during IVF treatment.

How long does acupuncture treatment last?

A typical acupuncture visit will last anywhere from 30 to 45 minutes depending on complexity, with the initial visit lasting as long as 1 1/2 hours (including examination and treatment). If the patient is considering IVF, acupuncture treatments will usually occur 1-2 times per week, with more frequent visits the week of retrieval and implantation. If trying to conceive naturally, an acupuncture course is usually once or twice per week for at least three to six months (or, if pregnancy is achieved, until end of first trimester). The patient will be re-evaluated periodically and may be encouraged to chart basal body temperature, cervical fluid, mood and menstrual symptoms to track changes.

I don't like needles. Is acupuncture painful?

This is an important question concerning those undergoing IVF, as the fear of needles will sooner or later have to be addressed. Many patients find acupuncture a good way to relieve their "needle- phobia" in preparation for their injections at the end of their IVF cycle. Acupuncture needles are the width of a human hair, and most patients will feel a sensation similar to a mosquito bite near the point site. Other areas, such as the feet and hands, are more sensitive but rarely bothersome. The effects of acupuncture usually result in relaxation or even a short nap during treatment.

My doctor diagnosed me with "unexplained infertility." Can acupuncture help?

Although no detectable abnormality is apparent, Chinese medicine often can detect a possible cause. By taking into account an array of symptoms presented from an Oriental medicine perspective, the correct acupuncture and Chinese medicinal protocol can be prescribed. In cases where the patient is motivated, healthy and compliant, the results are often good.

How do I know if my acupuncturist is qualified?

In order to practice acupuncture in the state of Florida, an acupuncturist must be licensed by the Florida Department of Health and board certified by the NCCAOM (National Certification Commission of Acupuncture and Oriental Medicine). Formal training at an accredited acupuncture school is completed in 3 1/2 to 4 years, in addition to at least 60 credit hours of undergraduate school beforehand. After graduation or during the last year of acupuncture training, the student can complete their training at affiliate hospitals in China. Check your state's guidelines at www.nccaom.org.

When choosing an acupuncturist, you may first want to inquire as to their main specialty before embarking on your acupuncture journey. Generally, an acupuncturist specializing in infertility is to be sought out, and many websites are devoted now to listing qualified practitioners by region. In 2008, a specialty board called the American Board of Oriental Reproductive Medicine (ABORM) was developed to ensure a higher standard of care for those patients undergoing Traditional Chinese Medicine treatment for infertility. Practitioners have passed a comprehensive exam in both Western and Eastern reproductive medicine in addition to completing additional courses pertaining to infertility. For a complete list of practitioners, go to www.aborm.org.

What other ways can acupuncture and herbal medicine help enhance fertility?

Acupuncture can help:
•Regulate menstrual cycles
•Regulate hormones to produce a better quality eggs and to produce a larger number of follicles during ART; decreasing FSH levels if elevated and increasing estrogen levels if these are low. •Increase implantation rates in IVF and IUI by 40%.
•Decrease uterine contractions, thus increasing implantation rates and decreasing the chance of miscarriage
•Increase blood flow to the reproductive organs and nourishing the thickness of the uterine lining
•Improve sperm quality and quantity

•Help to relieve the side effects of stimulation drugs during ART

•Easing stress, anxiety and depression, and promoting deep relaxation

What can I expect from treatment?

Clinically, conception rates are improved by 40% with the use of acupuncture and herbs. Many conditions may be alleviated very rapidly by acupuncture and herbal medicine. However, some conditions, which have arisen over a course of years will be relieved only with slower, steady progress. As in any form of healing, the patient's attitude, diet, determination and life-style will affect the outcome of a course of treatment. Patients are encouraged to actively participate in their healing process. The number of treatments you will need depends on your overall health, your body's response to acupuncture and/or Western reproductive treatments, and the nature and duration of your condition.

In my experience, I have found that both Western and Chinese medicine have strong, effective solutions to infertility and both systems of medicine have much to offer one another. As information grows about the benefits of Oriental medicine, it is important that patients develop a "team" of knowledgeable practitioners that understands the strengths and weaknesses of both systems and can help them along the often highly stressful road to fertility.

Chapter Ten: Arvigo™ Techniques of Mayan Abdominal Therapy (ATMAT)

Sylvia was an extremely busy professional in her mid 40's. She often complained of severe menstrual cramps due to endometriosis, for which a course of Chinese herbs and acupuncture had been prescribed. Every month, the pain improved gradually but Sylvia still admitted to taking over-the-counter pain relievers during her cycle. One afternoon, she walked into the clinic with a smile that lit up the entire treatment room. Sylvia was pain-free and felt amazing for the first time in her menstruating life. She had just returned from her first Arvigo Mayan abdominal therapy (ATMAT) session. Not only was Sylvia's cycle less painful, it was bright red and free of clotting. As she explained the treatment in more detail, I was intrigued. How could this therapy achieve results in such a short time? Acupuncture and Chinese herbs worked gradually, and we certainly did not expect to see results like this in one visit.

Sylvia described her session as a sort of "physical therapy" for her uterus. The therapist used gentle yet firm strokes on her lower abdomen just above her pubic bone, encouraging blood flow and healthy uterine positioning. She then moved up to her stomach to calm the digestion and finally, turning Sylvia over, she stretched and massaged the lower back and tailbone. Since the uterus is attached to the lower spine by several ligaments and nerve endings, her circulation and pain were improved after the first session. She was then taught a series of home self-care exercises to perform each night. Perhaps the most interesting part of the treatment was a traditional steam that Sylvia underwent with the therapist called a vaginal steam. Sylvia described it as feeling her entire body was warmed from inside. The therapist used herbs such as calendula, eucalyptus and lavender as part of the steam, and Sylvia draped herself with a blanket as she sat over a special stool with the center cut out. This allowed the steam to enter near the cervix and relax the perineal muscles.

I was intrigued, but was not fully convinced to investigate it further until three more patients came to the office after receiving treatment from the same therapist. The last one asked if I would undergo the training so she could combine it with her acupuncture sessions and I agreed. To this day, I am very appreciative of that patient, who became my first ATMAT patient and now has a healthy baby boy. Although Mayan abdominal therapy is practiced widely in Central America and Mexico, little is known about it in the United States. Research is currently underway to study the effects on infertility and dysmenorrhea (painful periods) from major universities. Ironically, we've had several patients who were referred by their grandmothers! They grew up massaging their bellies and wearing fajas, which are traditional wraps that fit snuggly around the waist to support the back and uterine ligaments after birth. As South Florida is a melting pot of cultures, we've even had patients from as far away as Morocco who were encouraged by their mothers to "get the uterus lifted."

They want their daughters and granddaughters to know this profound treatment that has been lost in the most recent generation of technology, drugs and surgery. After conducting our own research for the past year in the form of case studies submitted to the Arvigo Institute, we concluded that the majority of the women in our clinic requesting AMAT reported a drastic improvement in menstrual cramps, lower back pain, libido and cycle regulation. Almost all of these women had been diagnosed with endometriosis by their reproductive specialist and now were mostly asymptomatic. Those combining acupuncture and AMAT with IVF or IUI had higher pregnancy rates than those who were only treated with acupuncture.

We have now incorporated ATMAT into our treatment plans for women seeking pregnancy or with a history of painful menses. Interestingly, our findings indicate that most of the women diagnosed with infertility and endometriosis coming to our clinic also have a diagnosis of a retroverted or "tilted" uterus. Each session at our office is followed by a thirty-minute acupuncture treatment and infrared heat to the lower back or abdomen (depending on what stage of her cycle she is currently in.) After practicing ATMAT for one year, I was fortunate enough undergo advanced training with Dr. Rosita Arvigo, the founder of ATMAT and hear case studies from twenty other practitioners from around the globe who echoed my clinical experiences. Dr. Arvigo continues to teach ATMAT from her center in Belize and occasionally visits the United States to train advanced practitioners. For more information on this unique therapy and to locate a practitioner in your area, go to www.arvigotherapy.com. It is my hope that with further research this profound therapy can be provided alongside acupuncture in reproductive medicine clinics around the country one day.

Chapter Eleven:
Preparing for IVF/ IUI

After rounds of strenuous fertility testing, you and your partner are ready to take the plunge. If all of the planets align and your period comes as expected, then you will probably start a course of fertility medications at that time. If you have already done a course of acupuncture and possibly Chinese herbs consisting of 2-3 months of treatment, you will usually be recommended by your acupuncturist to increase the number of weekly treatments to 2-3 times per week during ovarian stimulation. This is particularly true if you have been labeled a "poor responder" by your fertility doctor or have just been referred for acupuncture without much prior treatment.

As we have discussed, laying the foundation of creating a healthy endometrium for the embryo(s) to implant is of utmost importance. By the time you start an IVF or IUI cycle, your acupuncturist would like to see that your menses have become more bright red and less clotty, and your hormones have normalized signaling a healthier response to the medications. In a nutshell, these are the suggestions that our patients follow:

• Emphasize increasing intake of fiber along with fresh organic fruits and vegetables to boost the liver's detoxifying capacity so that it is able to cope with the drugs that you will have to take during the treatment. Incorporating liver detoxifying herbs such as milk thistle or Liver GI Detox from Pure Encapsulations is also helpful when begun 3-6 months prior to starting a medicated cycle or trying naturally to conceive.

- Abstain from smoking and avoid smoky atmospheres: smoking damages the lining of the uterus and fallopian tubes, along with being detrimental to egg quality

- Try to avoid strenuous exercise, such as aerobics, or running. Your body needs rest as your hormonal system shuts down to prepare for IVF. Try gentle forms of exercise instead, such as walking or yoga.

- Avoid chocolate, sugary and processed foods, salty snacks, coffee, tea, cola and other carbonated drinks, and alcohol. These all counteract the beneficial effects of vital nutrients, and some have a diuretic effect.

- Drink at least 2 liters of filtered water a day. Water is vitally important for every cell in the body and to ensure the drugs you are taking during IVF go where they need to go in the body. Water is also important to prevent OHSS (ovarian hyperstimulation syndrome.)

- Eat about 60grams (2 oz) of protein a day. Insufficient protein in the diet can result in a reduced number of eggs.

- Undergo Arvigo Techiques of Maya Abdominal Therapy™ (ATMAT) 2-3 times per month if available to enhance blood flow and properly prepare the uterine lining.

Taking Supplements

If possible, start taking your nutritional supplements at least 3 to 4 months before your IVF treatment commences. I strongly advise that you ask your doctor or IVF nurse before taking any supplements. For those patients with abnormally elevated FSH levels, an interesting protocol of oral contraceptives, DHEA, L-arginine and acupuncture have been successful at "resetting" the pituitary in many of our patients and restoring hormonal balance. This protocol is recommended by several fertility clinics and has been an alternative to a donor egg cycle in patients who wish to try with their own eggs. We recommend Pure One by Pure Encapsulations for both partners which is a multivitamin high in antioxidants that contains the following:

-Vitamin B complex: will help your body cope with the stress of invasive procedures

-Vitamin C: 500 mg a day will help collagen production and is vital for wound healing following egg retrieval. There is some evidence to suggest that it may help to prevent miscarriage. Reduce Vitamin C intake to 250mg before transfer

-Vitamin E: enhances healing, improve fertilization rates (choose the natural version, known as d-alpha-tocopherol)

-Zinc: promotes cell formation and wound healing after surgery and is vital for hormone production and implantation, plays a vital role in cell division

-Selenium: improve fertilization rates, prevents chromosome breakage
-Magnesium: improve fertilization rates

-Folic Acid: prevents spina bifida, produce DNA and RNA. Some patients require a special form of folate called Metafolin which is more readily absorbed. -CoQ10: improve blood flow, enrich endometrium, may improve fertilization rates

-Myoinositol: Supports healthy mood and promotes healthy ovarian function. Some studies have shown it to improve egg quality as well.

-Essential Fatty Acids: (not found in Pure One) We recommend the brand Omaprem due to higher EFA concentration, improves blood viscosity, mood support

Other Tips:

-Arnica: this homeopathic remedy may help prevent bruising after injections, especially for those on blood thinners like Lovenox or baby Aspirin. Use topically after injections as a preventative measure if you are prone to bruising.

-Apply ice to numb the injection sites briefly prior to administering shots if you experience discomfort. -Use a hot water bottle to keep the abdomen warm and assist healing.

-Rest as much as you can in preparation for placing of the embryos in the uterus. Strenuous exercise during and following an IVF cycle is contraindicated and can have a negative effect of diverting blood flow away from the uterus in order to supply more vital organs such as the heart and lungs.

-Practice deep breathing and relaxation techniques to encourage good blood flow and energy around the body. There are several guided meditations available for download now online that specifically address the concerns of a medicated cycle. We use guided meditation for fertility (available at www.alunamoon.com) during acupuncture treatments at Florida Complete Wellness to enhance relaxation.

-After an embryo transfer, rest for a minimum of two days. Activity diverts blood to your extremities and vital organs, while lying down allows blood to flow to the endometrium. Especially if you have small children at home, try your best to recruit help at this time.

During the (approximate) two-week wait, just say no to:

• Caffeine, tobacco, alcohol, drugs

- Heavy lifting (over 15 lbs.)

- Strenuous exercise, including housework

- Bouncing activities, such as horseback riding

- Sun bathing, sauna, hot tubs, Jacuzzis, hot baths and swimming

- Sexual intercourse

After the embryo transfer, our clinic usually recommends to continue twice weekly acupuncture visits starting 4-5 days after the procedure and continuing until the pregnancy test. Research shows the stress and anxiety inherent in the 10-day wait period can be greatly reduced by receiving acupuncture and practicing relaxation strategies such as meditation or positive imagery. If the pregnancy test is positive, our patients continue their twice-weekly sessions until the ultrasound shows a heartbeat and they are mostly out of the "danger zone" of the first 6 weeks of pregnancy.

Chapter Twelve-Coping With A Failed IVF/IUI Cycle Or Miscarriage

Unfortunately, for some couples pregnancy remains elusive even after all of the preparation and hard work going into a cycle. What is the difference in pregnancy rates for couples with fertility problems between trying with regular intercourse versus IUI (intrauterine insemination?)

• A couple that has been trying for a year and a half and does not have tubal problems, sperm problems or endometriosis has about a 2-8% chance per month (over the next year) of getting pregnant from regular intercourse.

• If a similar couple combines Clomid with IUI's, the expected success rate is 10% per month for up to 3 months.

When methods such as acupuncture and mind-body approaches are incorporated, the odds are increased (as the research shows in the following chapter) and can possibly shorten the amount of medicated cycles the couple has to endure. Talking to a licensed psychologist specializing in infertility can be very beneficial as well. To locate one in your area, go to www.resolve.org and check under healthcare providers. To check the IVF success rates of your fertility clinic, go to www.sart.org and search by zip code. IVF success rates can vary widely from clinic to clinic, but know that you are not alone if the first, or second cycle does not succeed.

Failing an IVF or IUI cycle can be devastating. When faced with a pregnancy loss after a medicated cycle, the sadness and guilt can be overwhelming. "Maybe I should have rested more, not lifted anything, not had that argument with my mother-in-law, etc.." The truth is that nothing you did or didn't do caused this loss. Take time to grieve and heal without rushing into another cycle. Your hormone levels may take a while to normalize after IVF and especially after a miscarriage so be kind to yourself. It's okay to be angry and to acknowledge your grief. Your spouse or partner may or may not be as supportive as you'd hoped but reaching out to a support group or journaling about your feelings is an important step in the healing process.

If your miscarriage resulted in a D&C (dilation and curettage) procedure, you need to insist on a follow up ultrasound from your specialist to ensure that the process was 100% complete. Many times "products of conception" may be left behind and cause problems with menstrual cycle regulation and bleeding. Enduring a miscarriage is difficult enough, but not having a thorough D&C can prolong the devastation. We also recommend address any scar tissue that might have formed as a result of one or multiple D&C's with the use of natural enzymes taken after the procedure. Your acupuncturist can provide more information on this.

Although it may be hard to contemplate at this time, ask your doctor about testing the fetus for possible chromosome abnormalities. If the tests are normal, further tests may be needed to rule out possible immunological or autoimmune problems with you that may be preventing a healthy pregnancy. Diagnosing and treating the mother in very early pregnancy could prevent an alarming 50% of all recurrent miscarriages. This is done with a simple blood test that looks for factors such as blood clotting disorders and other autoimmune factors su ch as elevated natural killer cell activity that may be signaling the body to mistake the embryo for a foreign invader. Most of these tests can be performed with your fertility doctor or gynecologist.

A "fertility time out" (FTO) might be needed to heal from the constant stress of trying to conceive and only you and your partner will know how long this will be. Let your inner wisdom guide you to a correct resting place, and resume if and when you feel the time is right. Pressure from family, co-workers and friends can ultimately make or break your relationship with your partner if not addressed and the devastation of a failed cycle is often not fully understood by others who have not been fertility-challenged.

Chapter Thirteen: I'm Pregnant, Now What?

Congratulations, you've made it to the home stretch! If you've been trying naturally or have undergone an IUI prior to receiving a positive home pregnancy test, it's time to pay a visit to your reproductive specialist and share the good news. The most accurate way of confirming a pregnancy is through a blood test, which will detect the level of HCG pregnancy hormone in your body. If you have undergone an IVF cycle, your clinic will usually recommend holding off on a urine test and will schedule an appointment for an HCG blood test instead.

HCG stands for "Human Chorionic Gonadotropin", the pregnancy hormone that is produced by the placenta and enters the blood soon after implantation and is detected with pregnancy tests. HCG is being produced by the placenta and enters the blood stream as soon as implantation happens, about one week after fertilization and ovulation, when the embryo implants and the placenta attaches to the uterine lining.

What Do The Numbers Mean?

-hCG under 5mIU/ml: Negative,not pregnant

-hCG between 5-25 mIU/ml: "Equivocal". A low range that would need to be re-checked in a few days. Could be an indication of a late implantation or testing too early.

-hCG over 25 mIU/ml: You're pregnant!

You may be asked to return to your reproductive specialist every two days for repeat blood work to ensure your HCG levels are doubling. A single hCG reading is not enough information for most diagnoses. When there is a question regarding the health of the pregnancy, multiple testing of hCG done a couple of days apart gives a more accurate look at assessing the situation. After 2-3 adequate readings, you will be asked to return for an ultrasound in another week or two to confirm healthy fetal cardiac activity. Once fetal activity has been detected by ultrasound in a normal patient population, chances of normal delivery are about 95%.

There is a wide range of normal hCG levels and values and the values are different in blood serum or urine. Blood hCG levels are not very helpful to test for the viability of the pregnancy if the hCG level are above 6,000 and/or after 6-7 weeks of the pregnancy. Instead, to test the health of the pregnancy better, a sonogram should be done to confirm the presence of a fetal heartbeat. Once a fetal heart beat is seen, it is not recommended to check the pregnancy viability with hCG levels.

Urine hCG levels are usually lower than serum (blood) hCG levels. Blood hCG testing is much more sensitive than a urine HPT. This means that the blood test can detect pregnancy several days earlier than the urine test, as early as 2-3 days after implantation or 8-9 days after fertilization. Urine tests measure the urine HCG qualitatively, which means that the HPT results are either "positive" or "negative." Around the time of the first missed period (14+ days after ovulation), over 95% of HPTs are usually positive.

About 85% of normal pregnancies will have the hCG level double every 48-72 hours. As you get further along into pregnancy and the hCG level gets higher, the time it takes to double can increase to about every 96 hours. Caution must be used in making too much of hCG numbers. A normal pregnancy may have low hCG levels and deliver a perfectly healthy baby. The results on an ultrasound after 5 - 6 weeks gestation are much more accurate than using hCG numbers.

A transvaginal ultrasound should be able to see at least a gestational sac once the hCG levels have reached between 1,000 - 2,000mIU/ml. Because levels can differentiate so much and conception dating can be wrong, a diagnosis should not be made by ultrasound findings until the level has reached at least 2,000.

Implantation happens as early as 6 days after ovulation/fertilization (usually about 9 days after ovulation), so blood hCG can be found as early as 8-9 days after ovulation/fertilization. After an IVF transfer of a blastocyst embryo at day 5 or 6, implantation often happens within 24 hours. Pregnant women usually attain blood serum concentrations of at least 10-50 mIU/ cc in the 7-8 days following implantation.

If your blood HCG levels are not textbook perfect, take heart. Some normal pregnancies will have quite low levels of hCG and deliver perfectly healthy babies. Normal levels of hCG can vary tremendously. After 5-6 weeks of pregnancy, sonogram findings are much more predictive of pregnancy outcome than are HCG levels. Once the fetal heart rate is seen, most doctors will monitor the fetal heart rate rather than drawing more blood.

When is the right time to tell your family members and loved ones who have watched you and your partner struggle from the sidelines helplessly? That is a decision that you and your partner must decide on together before one of you posts a surprise comment on Facebook. For couples that have experienced a previous pregnancy loss, that time may come after the first trimester has passed uneventfully. For others, it may be after the first heartbeat is heard at the six-week ultrasound. The choice of when and who to tell is a very personal one, and often the right time is when both of you feel you can no longer keep it a secret!

Chapter Fourteen: Graduation Day

Although this day seemed like it would never come, you are officially leaving your fertility specialist and moving on to greener pastures. Ideally, you already have a gynecologist who also practices obstetrics and knows your case. If not, your fertility acupuncturist and/or reproductive endocrinologist can be a good source of referral. Most likely, they have worked with fertility- challenged women and will be open to collaborating with your reproductive endocrinologist during the transition if needed.

When To Say Goodbye

If you have gotten pregnant while undergoing acupuncture treatment, it is recommended to continue acupuncture until the end of the first trimester on a weekly basis after you have been referred to your obstetrician or midwife. After week 12-14, most patients are feeling more energetic and have gotten any nausea they might have experienced under control. At this time, acupuncture can be recommended as needed for back pain, heartburn, migraines or any other physical ailments that might crop up during pregnancy. Although most fertility acupuncturists have experience treating pregnant women, it's important to verify that your acupuncturist specializes in pregnancy as well. If he or she does not treat pregnant patients, ask for a referral.

On the other hand, if you conceived via ART (artificial reproductive technology) you will most likely be released after two consecutive ultrasounds have shown a viable pregnancy (or two!) The initial ultrasound is performed around two weeks after your initial pregnancy test is positive at 6 weeks. At this time, your reproductive endocrinologist will refer you to your obstetrician or midwife for care during the duration of your pregnancy. The visits to your obstetrician will be much less frequent than what you've been accustomed to at the fertility clinic, usually occurring only once per month until the end of the last trimester. Without constant monitoring, fears can crop up regarding the health of the pregnancy. Now is the time to ENJOY your pregnancy and release all of the stress that surrounded you and your partner while trying to conceive!

TIPS FOR REDUCING STRESS DURING PREGNANCY:

-Continue acupuncture and meditation

-Sleep seven to nine hours every night

-Share your concerns or problems with someone

-Recognize when you are stressed

-Exercise. Try swimming, walking or yoga

-Write down your feelings in a journal

-Limit strenuous activity and only do what you can handle

-Accept help. Let people know when you could use a hand.

-Connect with other moms and moms-to-be who have also experienced infertility by joining Facebook or Meetup groups in your area.

-Avoid stressful situations and people as much as possible.

Your journey has brought you to this much-anticipated day. After all of the appointments, injections, pills, and non-stop monitoring it may seem surreal when you receive the boot from your fertility clinic. You have overcome the odds and will be stronger as a couple and as parents-to-be for enduring the long months and even years of waiting. And although your patience may be tested, I hope this book has become your much-needed ally. You may reach me at fduro@floridacompletewellness.com and I welcome your comments or concerns. The best is yet to come.

Chapter Fifteen: Research on Acupuncture and IVF

Acupuncture and herbal medicine in in-vitro fertilization: a review of the evidence for clinical practice

Acupuncture and assisted conception

Cheong Y et al, Cochrane Database of Systematic Reviews 2009 Issue 1 Cochrane Database

A newer version of this database by the same authors as the one listed above concluded that there is an increase in live birth rate when acupuncture is performed on day of embryo transfer.

Abstract Background: Acupuncture has recently been studied in assisted reproductive treatment (ART) although its role in reproductive medicine is still debated. Objectives

To determine the effectiveness of acupuncture in the outcomes of ART. Search strategy

All reports which describe randomized controlled trials of acupuncture in assisted conception were obtained through searches of the Menstrual Disorders and Subfertility Group Specialized Register, CENTRAL, Ovid MEDLINE (1996 to August 2007), EMBASE (1980 to August 2007), CINAHL (Cumulative Index to Nursing & Allied Health Literature) (1982 to August 2007), AMED, National Research Register,Clinical Trials register(www.clinicaltrials.gov),and the Chinese database of clinical trials

Randomized controlled trials of acupuncture for couples who were undergoing ART comparing acupuncture treatment alone or acupuncture with concurrent ART versus no treatment, placebo or sham acupuncture plus ART for the treatment of primary and secondary infertility. Women with medical illness deemed contraindications for ART or acupuncture were excluded.

Data collection and analysis
Sixteen randomized controlled trials were identified that involved acupuncture and assisted conception. Thirteen trials were included in the review and three were excluded. Quality assessment and data extraction were performed independently by two review authors. Meta-analysis was performed using odds ratio (OR) for dichotomous outcomes. The outcome measures were live birth rate, clinical ongoing pregnancy rate, miscarriage rate, and any reported side effects of treatment.

Main results
There is evidence of benefit when acupuncture is performed on the day of embryo transfer (ET) on the live birth rate (OR 1.86, 95% CI 1.29 to 2.77) but not when it is performed two to three days after ET (OR 1.79, 95% CI 0.93 to 3.44). There is no evidence of benefit on pregnancy outcomes when acupuncture is performed around the time of oocyte retrieval.

Authors' conclusions

Acupuncture performed on the day of ET shows a beneficial effect on the live birth rate; however, with the present evidence this could be attributed to placebo effect and the small number of women included in the trials.

Effects of acupuncture on rates of pregnancy and live birth among women undergoing in vitro fertilization: systematic review and meta-analysis.

Manheimer E et al. BMJ 2008;336 pg 545-549 British Medical Journal

Early in 2008, the prestigious British Medical journal published its own analysis of the acupuncture in a meta-analysis of 7 of these trials; i.e. they chose only those which met strict research criteria.

The authors concluded, the odds ratio of 1.65 suggests that acupuncture increased the odds of clinical pregnancy by 65% compared with the control groups... In absolute terms 10 patients would need to be treated with acupuncture to bring about one additional clinical pregnancy. These are clinically relevant benefits.

And when they analyzed the 4 trials that measured live births in addition to pregnancy rates, they found that acupuncture increased the odds by 91% and that the number of patients who would need to be treated to bring about an additional pregnancy dropped to 9. Impressive as these results are they may still be an underestimate, since the authors included women whose IVF cycles were cancelled before transfer.

The accompanying editorial in the BMJ makes the comment that adding acupuncture to IVF improved pregnancy rates more than any other recent improvement or advance in IVF technology.

Abstract

Objective - To evaluate whether acupuncture improves rates of pregnancy and live birth when used as an adjuvant treatment to embryo transfer in women undergoing in vitro fertilization. Design - Systematic review and meta-analysis.

Data sources - Medline, Cochrane Central, Embase, Chinese Biomedical Database, hand-searched abstracts, and reference lists.

Review methods - Eligible studies were randomized controlled trials that compared needle acupuncture administered within one day of embryo transfer with sham acupuncture or no adjuvant treatment, with reported outcomes of at least one of clinical pregnancy, ongoing pregnancy, or live birth. Two reviewers independently agreed on eligibility; assessed methodological quality; and extracted outcome data. For all trials, investigators contributed additional data not included in the original publication (such as live births). Meta-analyses included all randomized patients.

Data synthesis - Seven trials with 1366 women undergoing in vitro fertilization were included in the meta-analyses. There was little clinical heterogeneity. Trials with sham acupuncture and no adjuvant treatment as controls were pooled for the primary analysis. Complementing the embryo transfer process with acupuncture was associated with significant and clinically relevant improvements in clinical pregnancy (odds ratio 1.65, 95% confidence interval 1.27 to 2.14; number needed to treat (NNT) 10 (7 to 17); seven trials), ongoing pregnancy (1.87, 1.40 to 2.49; NNT 9 (6 to 15); five trials), and live birth (1.91, 1.39 to 2.64; NNT 9 (6 to 17); four trials). Because we were unable to obtain outcome data on live births for three of the included trials, the pooled odds ratio for clinical pregnancy more accurately represents the true combined effect from these trials rather than the odds ratio for live birth.

The results were robust to sensitivity analyses on study validity variables. A prespecified subgroup analysis restricted to the three trials with the higher rates of clinical pregnancy in the control group, however, suggested a smaller non-significant benefit of acupuncture (odds ratio 1.24, 0.86 to 1.77).

Conclusions - **Current preliminary evidence suggests that acupuncture given with embryo transfer improves rates of pregnancy and live birth among women undergoing in-vitro fertilization.**

Traditional Chinese medicine and infertility

Huang, S T and Chen, A P C, Current Opinion in Obstetrics & Gynecology. 2008, 2(3):211-215. Current Opinion in Obstetrics & Gynecology

A recent review of current medical literature carried out by researchers in Taiwan noted that traditional Chinese medicine could regulate the gonadotropin- releasing hormone to induce ovulation and improve the uterus blood flow and menstrual changes of endometrium. In addition, it also has impacts on patients with infertility resulting from polycystic ovarian syndrome, anxiety, stress and immunological disorders. Their review concludes Integrating the principles and knowledge from well-characterized approaches and quality control of both traditional Chinese medicine and Western medical approaches should become a trend in existing clinical practice and serve as a better methodology for treating infertility.

Abstract

Purpose of review: The present review gives an overview of the potential use of traditional Chinese medicine in the treatment of infertility, including an evidence-based evaluation of its efficacy and tolerance.

Recent findings: Recent studies demonstrated that traditional Chinese medicine could regulate the gonadotropin-releasing hormone to induce ovulation and improve the uterus blood flow and menstrual changes of endometrium.

In addition, it also has impacts on patients with infertility resulting from polycystic ovarian syndrome, anxiety, stress and immunological disorders.

Although study design with adequate sample size and appropriate control for the use of traditional Chinese medicine is not sufficient, the effective studies have already indicated the necessity to explore the possible mechanisms, that is, effective dose, side effect and toxicity of traditional Chinese medicine, in the treatment of infertility by means of prospective randomized control trial.

Summary: The growing popularity of traditional Chinese medicine used alone or in combination with Western medicine highlights the need to examine the pros and cons of both Western and traditional Chinese medicine approaches. Integrating the principle and knowledge from well characterized approaches and quality control of both traditional Chinese medicine and Western medical techniques that will become a trend in existing clinical practice and serve as a better methodology for treating infertility.

Effect of acupuncture on the outcome of in vitro fertilization and intracytoplasmic sperm injection: a randomized, prospective, controlled clinical study

Dieterle S et al, Fertil Steril 2006 Vol 85, pg 1347-1351 Fertility and Sterility
Abstract
OBJECTIVE: To determine the effect of luteal-phase acupuncture on the outcome of IVF / intracytoplasmic sperm injection (ICSI).
DESIGN: Randomized, prospective, controlled clinical study.
SETTING: University IVF center.
PATIENT(S): Two hundred twenty-five infertile patients undergoing IVF/ICSI.
INTERVENTION(S): In group I, 116 patients received luteal-phase acupuncture according to the principles of traditional Chinese medicine. In group II, 109 patients received placebo acupuncture.

MAIN OUTCOME MEASURE(S): Clinical and ongoing pregnancy rates.

RESULT(S): In group I, the clinical pregnancy rate and ongoing pregnancy rate (33.6% and 28.4%, respectively) were significantly higher than in group II (15.6% and 13.8%).

CONCLUSION(S): **Luteal-phase acupuncture has a positive effect on the outcome of IVF/ICSI.**

Acupuncture: Impact on Pregnancy Outcomes in IVF Patients

12th World Congress on Human Reproduction, Venice Italy March 2005

Paul C. Magarelli, M.D., Ph.D. Reproductive Medicine & Fertility Center, Colorado Springs Diane Cridennda, L.Ac. East Winds Acupuncture Mel Cohen, MBA Reproductive Medicine & Fertility Center, Colorado Springs

Take Home babies' rates (THB) have been the sine quo non of IVF outcomes. Pregnancy rates (PR) can overestimate the expected success of a high-technology treatment for patients and many clinics use PR as means of marketing their practices. This has caused disillusionment in patients and government regulation (especially in the U.S.). Each IVF program strives to improve reproductive outcomes (low ectopic rates, low miscarriage rates and improved take home baby rates - live births).

Usually the approach to these improvements are changes in IVF protocols, media adjustments in the IVF lab, patient selection, and subtle nudges towards egg donors for poor responders. Another approach has been the inclusion of alternative medical modalities: acupuncture, massage therapy, stress reduction techniques, herbal medicine. We, and others, have chosen to incorporate Acupuncture into our IVF treatment protocols. Recently we presented two studies that demonstrated improvements in pregnancy rates in Good and Poor IVF Responders with the inclusion of two specific Acupuncture Protocols (Steiner- Victorin and Paulus et. Al). In the poor responders group we demonstrated a positive adjustment to Poor Responders pregnancy rates (PR) with improvements in PR in the Poor Responders group equivalent to good responders. In the Good Responders study we demonstrated a trend towards improved PR (5% above controls, not significant at $p < 0.05$). With these observations noted we have continued our investigation and are reporting on reproductive outcomes in all IVF patients treated with Acupuncture compared to those untreated.

Materials and Methods: In this study 130 IVF cycles were reviewed in a retrospective fashion. Patients demographics, years infertile, age of male partners, sperm parameters, Day 3 FSH, Pulsitility Indices, Weight, BMI, infertility diagnoses, IVF treatment protocols were statistically similar for both the Controls (C) and Acupuncture (Ac) treatment groups. All patients that completed an IVF cycle (retrieval, transfer) were included. There were 82 in the C group (non acupuncture) and 48 in the Ac group. For the C vs. Ac groups a summary of their statistics are as follows: Mean Age was 32.6 vs. 32.7, Day 3 FSH was 5.5 vs. 6.4, Pulsitility Indices for right and left uterine arteries were 1.5 and 1.2 vs. 1.4 and 1.0; Sperm counts were 69 vs. 67 million/ml; Sperm motility (%) were 48 vs. 53%, and Sperm morphologies were 6 % normal vs. 7%.

Results: Pregnancy rates for the Ac group were statistically similar, although numerically higher, versus C (50% v 45% at $P < 0.05$). Ac miscarriage rates (SAB) were statistically lower than the C (8 % vs. 11% at $p < 0.01$). There were no ectopic pregnancies in the Ac group ($P < 0.01$). Live Births were significantly better in the Ac v C groups (42% v 38%). A surprising observation was that multiples pregnancies were significantly lower in the Ac vs. C groups (17 % vs. 22%). Average eggs retrieved were statistically similar 15 vs. 15 for Ac and C respectively.

Conclusions: **IVF programs can significantly improve their IVF outcomes (PR, THB, SAB and Ectopic) by adding acupuncture protocols, specifically Steiner Victorin and Paulus.** Further studies of Traditional Chinese Medicine modalities of treatment are underway. We are organizing a multi-center prospective study to confirm our observations.

Acupuncture & IVF poor responders: a cure?

Magarelli P, Cridennda D, Fertil Steril, 2004; 81 Suppl 3 S20

Objective: The purpose of the study was to determine the influence of two acupuncture protocols on IVF outcomes and secondly to identify the appropriate patient groups that would most benefit from this adjunctive therapy.

Materials and Methods: In this retrospective study, data was extracted from medical records of patients RE&I clinic & acupuncture clinics between January 2001 and November 2003. All patients completing an IVF cycle with transfer were included. One RE&I provided the IVF care and a consortium of acupuncturists overseen by the author provided the strict acupuncture protocols. PR per transfer were the endpoints measured. Data was analyzed by student's t test and Multiregression with Wilcox ranking (MRW).

Results: 147 patients were included in the study and of those 53 had Acupuncture (Ac) and 94 did not (Non-Ac group). Demographic data between these Ac and Non-Ac groups respectively indicated remarkable equity (Table 1). Fertility Factors also demonstrated equity and there were no differences in Diagnoses, IVF Protocols and type of Gonadotropin protocols used.

Factors that demonstrated significance were: Length of time infertile, Peak FSH, PI for total group without MRW; PI for MRW groups reversed this (Table 2) and finally average: Sperm Morphology, Peak E2, Peak P4 prior to HCG: and endometrial thickness. PR before Wilcox ranking were the same: 40% v 38%. MRW analysis revealed FSH, Length of time trying to get pregnant, Sperm Morphology and E2 levels as significant: 6.5, 4.1, 4.0 and 1.6 respectively. When the Ac group was modified (15 Ac patient dropped), PI was elevated from 1.76 to 1.94 resulting in a significant elevation compared to the Non-Ac group, p 0.01. Also PR changed from 40% before to 53% after and this value was significantly greater than the Non-Ac group (38%), p 0.01.

Conclusions: **Significant increases in pregnancy outcomes were confirmed by this study and the data uniquely supported the advantage of acupuncture in patients with normal PI (prior studies were done on patient with PI).** We also demonstrated that both acupuncture treatment protocols could be used together with a synergistic effect. Finally, this study is the first to demonstrate that the use of acupuncture in patients with poor prognoses (elevated Peak FSH, longer history of infertility, poor sperm morphology) can achieve similar pregnancy rates to normal prognosis patients.

Acupuncture and Good Prognosis IVF Patients: Synergy

P. C. Magarelli, D. K. Cridennda, M. Cohen. Reproductive Medicine & Fertility Center, Colorado Springs, CO; East Winds Acupuncture, Inc., Colorado Springs, CO.

FERTILITY AND STERILITY®, Proceedings from the 2004 ASRM meeting in Philadelphia

OBJECTIVE: To determine the role of electro stimulation acupuncture and traditional combined with auricular acupuncture on IVF outcomes in good prognosis patients.

DESIGN: Retrospective case controlled clinical study. Acupuncture Consortium for treatment standardization. Reproductive Endocrinology & Infertility IVF Private Practice and Traditional Chinese Medicine Acupuncture Clinics.

MATERIALS AND METHODS: One hundred fourteen infertile patients undergoing controlled ovarian hyperstimulation with gonadotropins and GnRH agonist and antagonist for IVF-ET (2001 to 2003) in private practice IVF clinic. Only IVF patients with normal Day 3 FSH, normal uterine artery Pulsitility indices, sperm morphologies over 7% normal by Kruger Strict Criteria and good response to ovarian hyperstimulation protocols (i.e., E2 over 2000 pg/ml) were analyzed. Intervention (s): Electrostimulation acupuncture - reduction of Pulsitility Index (PI) of the uterine artery and Traditional combined with Auricular acupuncture - Pre/Post embryo transfer protocols were used alone or in combination and resultant pregnancy outcomes were measured after IVF treatments. Main Outcome Measure(s): Cycles were grouped according to those that received No Acupuncture (Non-Ac) and those that received either one or both acupuncture treatments (Ac).

Comparisons were made between Acupuncture treated IVF patients and Non-Acupuncture treated IVF patients in clinical pregnancies, ongoing pregnancies and birth outcomes. The statistics used for this analysis included; Tests for normal distribution: chi-square test, Kolmogorov-Smirnov Test Unpaired T-tests Stepwise Multiple regression Variance ratio test (F-Test) One-Way analysis of variance (ANOVA) with Student-Newman- Keuls (SNK) test for pair wise comparison of subgroups.

RESULTS: Total IVF cases 114, 53 with Acupuncture (Ac) and 61 without Acupuncture (Non-Ac). Demographics, Infertility Diagnoses, and Treatment Protocols were statistically the same between both groups and by design, the following parameters were similar: Sperm Morphology; Peak Day 3 FSH; Average Pulsitility Index; Peak E2 at hCG; and Post hCG P4. These parameters earned the designation of

Good Prognosis group. Pregnancy rates (PR) and Miscarriage rates (SAB) were statistically improved at the $p < 0.05$ levels in those patients that received Acupuncture (51% v 36% PR and 8% v 20% SAB in the AC v Non-Ac groups). There were no ectopic pregnancies in the Ac group and 9% in the Non-Ac group, $p < 0.008$.
Finally, Birth rates (BR) per cycle start and per pregnancy were significantly higher in the Ac group, with 23% more births/pregnancy significant at the $p < 0.05$ level.

CONCLUSION: The use of adjunctive therapies in IVF protocols is gaining popularity. In previously published data, Acupuncture was reserved for Poorer Prognosis patients and enhanced outcomes were observed. In this study, we demonstrated that Good Prognosis patients would also benefit from inclusion of published Acupuncture protocols. This is also the first publication of Birth outcome data in Acupuncture-treated IVF patients. **Acupuncture significantly increased birth outcomes it significantly decreased ectopic pregnancies and miscarriage rates.**These data uniquely support a definitive role of both Electrostimulation and Traditional combined with Auricular Acupuncture in IVF in Good Prognosis IVF patients.

Quintero R et al, Fertil Steril 2004 Vol 81 Suppl 3, pg S11-12 Fertility and Sterility

Abstract

Objective: The purpose of this study was to determine if there are benefits of standard acupuncture compared to sham acupuncture as an adjunct to IVF.

Materials and Methods: A randomized, controlled, double-blind, cross over pilot trial was performed using a needle-like device (sham acupuncture) as a control. Approval from GAMC's Investigational Review Board was acquired. Inclusion criteria were women aged 18 to

42 years with a history of failed IVF cycle(s); the presence of both ovaries; and a normal uterine cavity. Exclusion criteria was Kruger morphology <4%.

Results: Seventeen subjects were enrolled and seven subjects completed both arms of the study. The mean age was 36.2 years (range 28-41 years). The mean Day 3 FSH=3 D6.8 IU (range 3-13 IU). There were four ongoing pregnancies after the first cycle, equally distributed. Seven subjects were crossed over after the first cycle. Of these, four from the standard acupuncture group and one from the sham acupuncture group attained pregnancy. Two subjects of the standard acupuncture group were on-going pregnancies and one from the sham group. Only the sham group had two IVF cancellations. An unpaired Mann-Whitney Test using a two-sided p value was performed.

Conclusions: **Our study shows a significantly lower amount of gonadotropins used when IVF is combined with standard acupuncture. A 70% pregnancy rate was also achieved with standard acupuncture and IVF, compared to 25%. Larger prospective trials are necessary.**

Reduction of blood flow impedance in the uterine arteries of infertile women with electro-acupuncture.

Hum Reprod. 1996 Jun;11(6):1314-7.
Stener-Victorin E, Waldenström U, Andersson SA, Wikland M.
Department of Obstetrics and Gynaecology, Fertility Centre Scandinavia, University of Gothenburg, S-413 45 Gothenburg, Sweden.

Abstract
In order to assess whether electro-acupuncture (EA) can reduce a high uterine artery blood flow impedance, 10 infertile but otherwise healthy

women with a Pulsitility index (PI) >=3.0 in the uterine arteries were treated with EA in a prospective, non-randomized study. Before inclusion in the study and throughout the entire study period, the women were down-regulated with a gonadotrophin-releasing hormone analogue (GnRHa) in order to exclude any fluctuating endogenous hormone effects on the PI. The baseline PI was measured when the serum oestradiol was <=0.1 nmol/l, and thereafter the women were given EA eight times, twice a week for 4 weeks. The PI was measured again closely after the eighth EA treatment, and once more 10-14 days after the EA period. Skin temperature on the forehead (STFH) and in the lumbosacral area (STLS) was measured during the first, fifth and eighth EA treatments. Compared to the mean baseline PI, the mean PI was significantly reduced both shortly after the eighth EA treatment (P < 0.0001) and 10-14 days after the EA period (P < 0.0001). STFH increased significantly during the EA treatments. It is suggested that both of these effects are due to a central inhibition of the sympathetic activity. **In anovulatory infertility cases the hyperactive sympathetic system can be depressed by electro-acupuncture and the function of the hypothalamus-pituitary-ovarian axis can be regulated by electro acupuncture via central sympathetic system**

Use of Acupuncture before and after embryo transfer

Dalton-Brewer N et al, Hum Fert 2010 Vol 12 No 4 212 - 255
Human Fertility (abstracts from UK Fertility Societies Conference 2009)

This report describes outcomes for all patients who attended the London Bridge Fertility, Gynaecology and Genetics Centre in London over a two-year period and who had acupuncture. In the acupuncture group positive pregnancy rates/ET were 44.6% comparing favorably with the non-acupuncture historic control group. When they analyzed outcomes in different age groups they discovered that acupuncture intervention was particularly effective in woman in the 35-39 and the over 40 group.

Abstract

Use of Acupuncture before and after embryo transfer

Nick Dalton-Brewer, David Gillott,Nataly Atalla, Mohamed Menabawey, Pauline Wright,&Alan Thornhill
The London Bridge Fertility, Gynaecology and Genetics Centre, London, UK

All IVF cases in which acupuncture was administered before and after embryo transfer at a large private infertility centre were reviewed for a 2 year period. All patients were treated by the same practitioner (NDB) using Traditional Chinese Acupuncture (TCA). Patients received acupuncture to the protocol developed by Paulus, W.E., Zhang, M., Strehler, E., El-Danasouri, I., & Sterzik, K. (2002). Influence of acupuncture on the pregnancy rate in patients who undergo assisted reproduction therapy. Fertility & Sterility, 77, 721–724: Liver 3, Spleen 8, Stomach 29, Pericardium 6, GV 20 were manually stimulated five times over a 40-min period, at Bridge, approximately 10–20 minutes prior to embryo transfer. Embryo transfer was carried out under ultrasound guidance as per routine at Bridge. Ten minutes following embryo transfer acupoints Spleen 6, Stomach 36, Spleen 10, Large Intestine 4 were manually stimulated five times over a 40-min period before discharging the patient. Ear points 34, 55 and 58 were used in both treatments and not stimulated. A total of 71 patients underwent 74 cycles involving acupuncture before and after embryo transfer.
Overall, positive pregnancy rates/ET were 44.6% comparing favorably with the non-acupuncture historic control group.

When analyzed by maternal age at time of treatment, biochemical pregnancy results for acupuncture treated women were as follows: <35 years–52%; 35–39 years – 45%; 40–45 years – 35%.

Results for women aged 35–39 years and those over 40 years were markedly better than controls suggesting that acupuncture intervention of this type may be more effective in older women. No side effects or complications were experienced by women receiving acupuncture. Acupuncture is a safe, adjunct therapy in IVF and in other randomized clinical trials has been shown to significantly improve outcomes when used at the IVF centre before and after embryo transfer. Our preliminary data are encouraging and suggest that a trial involving older women may be effective.

The relationship between perceived stress, acupuncture, and pregnancy rates among IVF patients: A pilot study

Balk J et al, Compl Therapies in Clinical Practice 2010,16,154–157 Complementary Therapies in Clinical Practice

These researchers at a university IVF clinic in Pittsburgh were interested to investigate the relationship between acupuncture, stress and pregnancy rates. **The patients who received acupuncture on the day of embryo of transfer had a pregnancy rate of 55.6% compared with the control group pregnancy rate of 35.5%.**

Abstract

The aim of this paper was to determine the effect of acupuncture on perceived stress levels in women on the day of embryo transfer (ET), and to determine if perceived stress levels at embryo transfer correlated with pregnancy rates. The study was an observational, prospective, cohort study based at the University IVF center.

Patient(s): 57 infertile patients undergoing IVF or IVF/ICSI. Interventions(s): Patients were undergoing Embryo Transfer with or without acupuncture as part of their standard clinical care. Main outcome measure(s): Perceive Stress Scale scores, pregnancy rates.

Result(s): women who received this acupuncture regimen achieved pregnancy 64.7%, whereas those without acupuncture achieved pregnancy 42.5%. When stratified by donor recipient status, only non-donor recipients potentially had an improvement with acupuncture (35.5% without acupuncture vs. 55.6% with acupuncture). Those who received this acupuncture regimen had lower stress scores both pre-ET and post-ET compared to those who did not. Those with decreased perceived stress scores compared to baseline had higher pregnancy rates than those who did not demonstrate this decrease, regardless of acupuncture status.

Conclusions(s): **The acupuncture regimen was associated with less stress both before and after embryo transfer, and it possibly improved pregnancy rates. Lower perceived stress at the time of embryo transfer may play a role in an improved pregnancy rate.**

Acupuncture performed before and after embryo transfer improves pregnancy rates

Youran D et al Fertil Steril 2008 Vol. 90, Suppl 1, pg S240 Fertility and Sterility
Abstract
OBJECTIVE: Conflicting evidence exists on whether acupuncture is beneficial for patients undergoing In Vitro Fertilization (IVF) cycles. Therefore, this study was undertaken to determine whether on-site acupuncture, performed both before and after embryo transfer, affects clinical outcomes.

DESIGN: Retrospective data analysis.

MATERIALS AND METHODS: The Acupuncture Group consisted of 49 patients who received acupuncture on-site before and after embryo transfer in 2007. The treatment did not follow the Paulus protocol. The Control Group was 212 patients with no acupuncture undergoing IVF cycles in the same time period. The data was subdivided by SART age classifications to determine if acupuncture differentially benefitted certain age groups. Clinical Pregnancy Rate (CPR) was defined as the presence of fetal cardiac activity. Loss Rate was the percentage of pregnancies that did not proceed from a positive hCG to a clinical pregnancy. Data were analyzed using the unpaired t-test and Fisher's exact test, with significance defined as $P < 0.05$.

RESULTS: Patients with a positive hCG were significantly higher in the Acupuncture Group for women less than 35 years old (63.3% vs. 43.2%, p 1/4 0.048). The Acupuncture Group also had a higher CPR in the under 35 category (60.0% vs. 34.6%, p 1/4 0.01). There were no differences in the other age groups. Combining all the age groups, the cycle parameters between the two Groups were equivalent, while the CPR was higher and the Loss Rate lower for the Acupuncture group (Table 1).

TABLE 1. Cycle Data for All Age Groups Acupuncture No Acupuncture P Value

Age 32.6 +4.2 32.0 + 3.8 0.33
No. Oocytes 13.7 + 6.6 13.2 +6.9 0.65 22
Cell Number 6.8 + 2.0 7.0 + 2.1 0.36
Fragmentation Score 2.5 + 0.6 2.5 + 0.6 1.00
No. Embryos Frozen 2.5 + 3.2 2.7 + 3.5 0.85
No. Embryos Transferred 2.3 + 0.6 2.2 + 0.6 0.29 Positive hCG (%) 57.1 (28/49) 45.8 (97/212) 0.16 Clinical Pregnancy (%) 55.1 (27/49) 34.4 (75/212) 0.01 Loss Rate (%) 3.6 (1/28) 22.7 (22/97) 0.02

CONCLUSIONS: **Although other studies regarding acupuncture have been inconclusive, perhaps these positive results are related to two important factors. The treatments were performed on-site, eliminating the stress of traveling to another site before and after the embryo transfer. Also, the acupuncture treatment protocol did** not follow the traditional **Paulus protocol, thereby suggesting there is still more research to be done on how best to treat infertility issues with acupuncture.**

Laser acupuncture before and after embryo transfer improves ART delivery rates.

Fratterelli JL et al Fertil Steril 2008 Vol 90, Suppl 1,pg S105 Fertility and Sterility Abstract

This study reports an increase in implantation rates with the use of laser acupuncture however the overall pregnancy rates for laser or needle acupuncture were not significantly different to control groups. The control groups in this trial had a high clinical pregnancy rate i.e. over 50%.

DESIGN: Prospect randomized double blind and placebo controlled.

MATERIALS AND METHODS: On the day of transfer, participants were randomly assigned to a study group; needle acupuncture (AC), laser acupuncture (LZ AC), sham laser acupuncture (LZ sham), relaxation (RX), or no treatment (NT). The AC and LZ AC puncture groups were considered treatment groups, the RX controls for the additional rest before and after transfer, and NT is the non-intervention group. Most significantly, the LZ Sham group provided an important control group. The laser acupuncture device was randomly preprogrammed per case to either fire (and provide LZ AC) or to not fire and thus provide a true double blind control group (LZ sham). It was not possible for the patient or acupuncturist to know if the laser fired. No contact occurs with the patient in laser acupuncture so there is no acupressure effect or contact with the wrong meridians. All treatments were administered for 25 minutes before and after embryo transfer. Outcomes were compared by Chi-square and multiple logistic regression analysis to control for the potential confounders including female age, embryo quality, and day of transfer (Table 1).

RESULTS: All treatments were well tolerated. No differences in terms of patient demographics, cycle type, stimulation outcomes, embryo number and quality, day of embryo transfer, transferring physician, or acupuncturist were found between the 5 study groups. Implantation rates were significantly improved with laser acupuncture. Traditional needle acupuncture had outcomes equivalent to the 3 control groups. Sub analyses of patient age and embryo transfer day produced similar findings with laser acupuncture enhancing outcome rates.

CONCLUSIONS: **This large prospective randomized and well-controlled study consistently demonstrated benefit to laser acupuncture. Treatment was well tolerated and significantly improved implantation rates.**

Table 1.

Clinical Outcomes (%) Rates

AC LZ AC LZ Sham RX NT P Values Impl 28.9 33.7 26.8 24.9 30.2 < 0.05

Chem Preg 61.5 60.9 53.0 53.7 60.4 0.22 Clin Preg 51.5 54.5 43.9 45.3 50.3 0.19

Cont Preg 39.0 42.1 35.4 37.4 39.6 0.71

The effect of acupuncture on outcomes in in-vitro fertilization (IVF)

Udoff L. C. et al, Fertil Steril 2007 Vol 86, Issue 3, pg S145 Fertility and Sterility

OBJECTIVE: To develop a protocol that could be used in future studies to evaluate whether acupuncture improves pregnancy and delivery rates in patients undergoing IVF. DESIGN: Randomized, sham treatment controlled pilot study.

MATERIALS AND METHODS: Patients planning to undergo IVF who meet inclusion/exclusion criteria (age 40 years old at start of stimulation, highest basal FSH 10mIU/mL, 3 prior failed IVF attempts, acupuncture naive) were randomly assigned to an acupuncture treatment group or a sham treatment group.

Treatment sessions occurred before the start of gonadotropin stimulation, the day before the oocyte retrieval, the day before the embryo transfer and the day after the embryo transfer.

Acupuncture was performed using manual manipulation at 6 to 10 points depending on the timing of the acupuncture treatment. Sham treated patients had needles placed in non-meridian points at a shallow depth. Patients were also given a questionnaire regarding their impressions of acupuncture treatment and were asked to guess their group assignment.

Data was analyzed using chi-squared for dichotomous outcome variables (e.g. clinical pregnancy rate, number of take home babies) and t-tests for continuous outcomes (e.g. age).

RESULTS: Twenty-two IVF cycles (19 patients) were randomized with thirteen patients completing the study (14 cycles). Five cycles were not completed due to poor response to ovarian stimulation (4 in the sham group, one in the real group). Other reasons for incomplete cycles (all in the sham group) included a persistent ovarian cyst, no viable embryos for transfer and personal reasons. The overall cycle cancellation rate was 32% compared to a 22% cycle cancellation rate for non-study patients of a similar age treated at this center during a similar time period (p.05).

In the 13 patients analyzed, the mean age was 35 years old (SD4.03). There was no statistical difference between true and sham acupuncture groups with respect to age (Sham: Mean35, SD4.6, Real: Mean34, SD4.6). Additionally, there was no significant difference between groups in highest basal FSH, number of oocytes retrieved, or number of embryos transferred. There was a significantly higher chemical pregnancy rate (80% versus 11.0%) in patients receiving true acupuncture compared to sham acupuncture (p.05). **The clinical pregnancy rates and the take home baby rates showed a strong trend towards a higher rate with acupuncture treatment though the difference was not statistically significant (60% real treatment vs. 11% sham treatment, p.05.).**

Regarding the questionnaire, only one patient correctly guessed their group assignment (real acupuncture). All patients rated their experience as very positive or positive.

CONCLUSION: It is feasible to conduct a randomized, blinded, sham control trial to study the impact of acupuncture on IVF success rates. Such a protocol is well accepted by patients.

Preliminary data shows a statistically significant improvement in the biochemical pregnancy rate with acupuncture treatment. Additionally, acupuncture was associated with a strong trend towards higher clinical pregnancy rates and take home baby rates, though more patients will need to be studied to reach any final conclusions.

The effect of acupuncture in assisted reproduction techniques

Teshima D. R. K et al, Fertil Steril 2007 Vol 88, Suppl 1, pg S330
Fertility and Sterility Abstract

OBJECTIVE: The aim of this study was to evaluate the effects of acupuncture on embryo transfer by comparing the rates of clinical pregnancy. 25 DESIGN: Retrospective, interventional and longitudinal study.

MATERIALS AND METHODS: Study with a total of 111 cycles of patients who underwent assisted reproduction techniques: in vitro fertilization (IVF) or intracytoplasmic sperm injection (ICSI) from June/2005 to January/ 2007: 52 cycles with acupuncture and 59 cycles without acupuncture. Acupuncture was performed, in specific points of the body including the ear, immediately before and after the embryo transfer procedure and the needles were retained for 30 minutes per session. The embryo transfer was carried out under ultrasound guidance and luteal phase sup- port was given by trans-vaginal progesterone administration (Utrogestan) and intramuscular progesterone. Outcome measure was clinical pregnancy rate.

RESULTS: The clinical pregnancy rate per cycle was observed in 27 of 52 (51.9%) patients in the acupuncture group and 21 of 59 (35.6%) patients in the control group (P 1/40,083). The mean age was 36.1 6.1 years in the control group and 36.4 years in the acupuncture group (P1/40.785). The mean number of embryo transferred was 3.3 in the control group and 3.6 in the acupuncture group (P1/40.462). The technique of embryo transfer was 5 cycles of IVF and 54 cycles of ICSI in the control group and 5 cycles IVF and 47 cycles of ICSI in the acupuncture group (P 1/41.000). Both groups did not show statistics difference in the mean age, number of embryo transferred and the technique procedure.

CONCLUSIONS: **Although there was a higher pregnancy rate in the acupuncture group, this difference was not statistically** significant, probably because of the small number of patients in

both group. Acupuncture seems to be an important co-adjutant in the treatment of infertility with IVF or ICSI, and further research is needed to demonstrate its precise effect.

Acupuncture in IVF Linked to Lower Miscarriage and Ectopic Rates

Cridennda Diane K, Magarelli Paul, Cohen Mel Research Presented at ASRM 2007

PHILADELPHIA - **Women who receive acupuncture during the stimulation phase of an in vitro fertilization cycle and again immediately after embryo transfer have a higher live-birth rate than do controls, according to the first acupuncture study with this end point.**

"Other studies have looked at pregnancy rates, but what is really important is whether or not there is a baby," said Paul C. Magarelli, M.D., who reported his findings at the annual meeting of the American Society for Reproductive Medicine.

The retrospective study included 131 women who were undergoing standard in vitro fertilization (IVF) or Intracytoplasmic sperm injection (ICSI). All of these women were considered good prognosis candidates for IVF/ICSI and were given the choice of having acupuncture. A total of 83 women declined (controls) and 48 accepted. There were no significant differences between the two groups in terms of infertility diagnoses, demographics, and treatment protocols, except that sperm morphology was slightly better in the partners of women receiving acupuncture (7.3% vs. 5.9 % normal forms with strict criteria evaluation), and the average uterine artery Pulsitility index was lower in the acupuncture group (1.57 vs. 1.72), said Dr. Magarelli .

"The live-birth rate per pregnancy is an even more telling number, since some cycles get cancelled. There was a 42% live-birth rate per pregnancy in the acupuncture group, compared to a 35% rate in the non-acupuncture group," Dr. Magarelli said in an interview with this newspaper. —We believe that what we are doing is improving the uterine environment such that implantation is improved," he added. The study used two acupuncture protocols. The Stener-Victorin electro stimulation protocol-which has been shown to reduce high uterine artery blood flow impedance, or Pulsitility index (Hum. Reprod. 1996;11:1314-7)-was used for nine treatments during ovarian stimulation. The second acupuncture technique-the Paulus protocol, which has been associated with improved pregnancy rates (Fertil. Steril. 2002; 77:721-4)-was used within 24 hours before the embryo transfer and 1 hour after.

Acupuncture and IVF embryo transfer, ART and PCOS

Acupuncture Med. 2006 Dec;24(4):157-63.
Use of acupuncture in female infertility and a summary of recent acupuncture studies related to embryo transfer.
Stener-Victorin E, Humaidan P.
Institute of Neuroscience and Physiology, Sahlgrenska Academy, Goteborg University, Sweden. elisabet.stener-victorin@neuro.gu.se

During the last five years the use of acupuncture in female infertility as an adjuvant to conventional treatment in assisted reproductive technology (ART) has increased in popularity. The present paper briefly discusses clinical and experimental data on the effect of acupuncture on uterine and ovarian blood flow, as an analgesic method during ART, and on endocrine and metabolic disturbances such as polycystic ovary syndrome (PCOS). Further it gives a summary of recent studies evaluating the effect of acupuncture before and after embryo transfer on pregnancy outcome.

Of the four published RCTs, three reveal significantly higher pregnancy rates in the acupuncture groups compared with the control groups. But the use of different study protocols makes it difficult to draw definitive conclusions. It seems however, that acupuncture has a positive effect and no adverse effects on pregnancy outcome.

Influence of acupuncture stimulation on pregnancy rates for women undergoing embryo transfer

Smith C et al, Fertil Steril 2006 Vol 85, pg 1352-1358 Fertility and Sterility

Abstract

OBJECTIVE: To evaluate the effects of acupuncture on clinical pregnancy rates for women undergoing ET.

DESIGN: Single-blind, randomized controlled trial using a noninvasive sham acupuncture control.

SETTING: Repromed, The Reproductive Medicine Unit of The University of Adelaide.

PATIENT(S): Women undergoing IVF.

INTERVENTION(S): Women were randomly allocated to acupuncture or noninvasive sham acupuncture with the placebo needle. All women received three sessions, the first undertaken on day 9 of stimulating injections, the second before ET, and the third immediately after ET.

MAIN OUTCOME MEASURE(S): The primary outcome was pregnancy. Secondary outcomes were implantation, ongoing pregnancy rate at 18 weeks, adverse events, and health status.

RESULT(S): Two hundred twenty-eight subjects were randomized. The pregnancy rate was 31% in the acupuncture group and 23% in the control group. For those subjects receiving acupuncture, the odds of achieving a pregnancy were 1.5 higher than for the control group, but the difference did not reach statistical significance. The ongoing pregnancy rate at 18 weeks was higher in the treatment group (28% vs. 18%), but the difference was not statistically significant.

CONCLUSION(S): **There was no significant difference in the pregnancy rate between groups; however, a smaller treatment effect cannot be excluded. Our results suggest that acupuncture was safe for women undergoing ET.**

Acupuncture on the day of embryo transfer significantly improves the reproductive outcome in infertile women: a prospective, randomized trial

Westergaard L et al, Fertil Steril 2006 Vol 85, pg 1341-1346 Fertility and Sterility Abstract

OBJECTIVE: To evaluate the effect of acupuncture on reproductive outcome in patients treated with IVF/intracytoplasmic sperm injection (ICSI). One group of patients received acupuncture on the day of ET, another group on ET day and again 2 days later (i.e., closer to implantation day), and both groups were compared with a control group that did not receive acupuncture.

DESIGN: Prospective, randomized trial. SETTING: Private fertility center.

PATIENT(S): During the study period all patients receiving IVF or ICSI treatment were offered participation in the study. On the day of oocyte retrieval, patients were randomly allocated (with sealed envelopes) to receive acupuncture on the day of ET (ACU 1 group, n = 95), on that day and again 2 days later (ACU 2 group, n = 91), or no acupuncture (control group, n = 87).

INTERVENTION(S): Acupuncture was performed immediately before and after ET (ACU 1 and 2 groups), with each session lasting 25 minutes; and one 25-minute session was performed 2 days later in the ACU 2 group.

MAIN OUTCOME MEASURE(S): Clinical pregnancy and ongoing pregnancy rates in the three groups.

RESULT(S): **Clinical and ongoing pregnancy rates were significantly higher in the ACU 1 group as compared with controls (37 of 95 [39%] vs. 21 of 87 [26%] and 34 of 95 [36%] vs. 19 of 87 [22%]).**

Impact of acupuncture before and after embryo transfer on the outcome of in vitro fertilization cycles: A prospective single blind randomized study

Benson M. R. et al, Fertil Steril 2006 Vol 86, Issue 3, pg S135 Fertility and Sterility Abstract

OBJECTIVE: The study was conducted to examine several adjunct treatment regimens administered before and after embryo transfer and determine if one treatment was more efficacious than any of the alternative regimens on in vitro fertilization (IVF) outcome. We compared two different acupuncture stimulation modes, needle and laser acupuncture, with sham laser acupuncture, relaxation, or no intervention treatment on implantation and pregnancy rates in women undergoing IVF.

DESIGN: Prospective single blind randomized trial. MATERIALS AND METHODS: Patients (n258) who had been scheduled for embryo transfer (ET), signed informed consent and were randomly assigned to one of 5 study treatment regimens; needle acupuncture (AC; 53), laser acupuncture (LZ AC; n53), sham laser acupuncture (placebo)(LZ sham; n52), relaxation (RX; n50), or no intervention treatment (NT; n50). All treatments were administered 25 minutes before ET and immediately after ET. The patient and acupuncturist were unaware of whether the laser system was active which allowed for a double-blind control group for the laser acupuncture treatment. Comparisons of various parameters between groups were conducted by 2 tests and one-way ANO- As.. Multinomial logistic regression analysis was used to control for the potentially confounding effects of day of embryo transfer (day 3 vs.5) and number of embryos transferred which are known to relate to IVF outcome, to further analyze the impact of adjunct treatment regimens on implantation and pregnancy rates. Probability of P 0.05 was considered to be statistically significant.

ACU 2 group (36% and 26%) were higher than in controls, but the difference did not reach statistical difference.

CONCLUSION(S): **Acupuncture on the day of ET significantly improves the reproductive outcome of IVF/ICSI, compared with no acupuncture. Repeating acupuncture on ET day +2 provided no additional beneficial effect.**

Improvement of IVF Outcomes by Acupuncture: Are egg and embryo qualities involved? Paul C. Magarelli, M.D., Ph.D., a Diane Cridennda, L.Ac. b, Mel Cohen, MBA

FERTILITY AND STERILITY®, May 2005, VOL 83, SUP 2, Proceeding from the 2005 Pacific Coast Reproductive Society annual meeting in Palm Springs

Objective: In this study, we examine the impact of Acupuncture on the embryology characteristics of IVF patients, i.e., are there changes in the numbers of eggs generated, embryos fertilized, embryos transferred or remaining embryos for freezing in those patients receiving acupuncture therapy.

Design: Retrospective clinical study

Setting: Private infertility practice and Traditional Chinese Medicine practice

Patients: Two hundred eight IVF cycles were reviewed, 95 received acupuncture (Ac) and 113 were controls (C).

Interventions: Patients randomly chose Ac to complement their IVF treatments. Two published Ac protocols were used. Standard IVF protocols were used and done in one clinic by one physician. The MD was not aware of who received Ac in addition to their IVF. After three years the data were collected and analyzed.

Main Outcome Measures: Number of eggs retrieved, number of eggs fertilized normally, number of embryos implanted, number of embryos frozen, number of embryos transferred, day of transfer, number of prior IVF cycles, Day 3 FSH, Pulsitility Indices, weight, infertility diagnoses, IVF treatment protocols, pregnancy rates, SAB rates, ectopic rates, and multiple pregnancy rates.

Results: Number of prior IVF cycles, Day 3 FSH, Pulsitility Indices, Weight, Infertility diagnoses, IVF treatment protocols were statistically similar. Pregnancy rates for the Ac group were statistically significantly higher than the C group ($P \leq 0.05$), SAB rates were lower and multiple pregnancy rates were lower ($P < 0.06$, not statistically significant). Ectopic pregnancy rates were statistically lower in the Ac group ($P \leq 0.05$). There were no statistically significant differences between the C and Ac treated groups for the following embryology parameters: number of eggs retrieved, number of eggs fertilized normally, number of embryos implanted, number of embryos frozen, number of embryos transferred, and day of transfer.

Conclusions: **There were no discernable statistical differences between embryology characteristics in patients treated with or without Acupuncture. These data suggests that the mechanism of action of Acupuncture on IVF outcomes may be related to affects in the host (the egg provider and the embryo recipient) rather than in direct changes to the eggs retrieved and the embryos created.**

Acupuncture and In Vitro Fertilization: Does the Number of Treatments Impact Reproductive Outcome?

D.K. Cridennda L.Ac.(1), P.C. Magarelli MD, Ph.D. (2) , and M. Cohen, MBA (2).
(1), East Winds Acupuncture Colorado Springs, CO; (2) Reproductive Medicine & Fertility Center, Colorado Springs, CO

Objective: The purpose of this study was to determine the optimal number of acupuncture treatments that provide the patient with the best IVF outcomes, i.e., pregnancy.

Materials and Methods: Retrospective clinical study in private practice Acupuncture and IVF center. Data were compiled in a group of infertile patients (n = 216) who received acupuncture during their IVF treatment cycle between 2001 and 2005. Data were analyzed to determine the optimal number of Electrical Stimulation (e-Stim) acupuncture treatments (Stener-Victorin protocol) that would result in a clinical pregnancy.

Two hundred sixteen patients over a 4-year period were included in this study. Based on our previous studies, we determined a significant improvement in IVF outcomes when patients were treated with Acupuncture (Ac). We utilized two protocols: Stener-Victorin et al 1996 (reported on uterine blood flow) and Paulus et al. 2002 protocol (reported on acupuncture given just before and just after embryo transfer). Patients received a combination of both protocols. This population was stratified into pregnant and non- pregnant groups and then evaluated by Student T=test and Chi-Square analysis for age, FSH levels, weight, BMI and E-2 levels. The pregnant and non-pregnant groups were further subdivided into those that received or did not receive acupuncture and were analyzed by Chi-square analysis. Since all patients received acupuncture consisting of e-Stim, their distribution was analyzed utilizing Kaplan- Meier survival analysis for pregnancy and no pregnancy to determine the number of e-stimulation that would provide the greatest chance for pregnancy.

Results: Patients age, day 3 FSH levels, weight, BMI (body mass index) and E2 (estrogen level at embryo transfer) were not statistically significantly different between the Non Acupuncture (No Ac) and the Acupuncture (Ac) groups. There was a statistically significant improvement ($p < 0.01$) in pregnancy rates in the group that received Ac (49 patients of 106 (37.4%) in the No Ac became pregnant vs. 77 patients of 111 (61.1%) of the Ac group became pregnant). This is over 23% increase in pregnancy rates in the Ac group. When the data were compared between e- Stim treatments in the Ac only group, an average of 6.5 treatments were found in the non-pregnant Ac group and 5.9 treatments in pregnant Ac group (not statistically significantly different). When the data were plotted comparing pregnant vs. non-pregnant Ac patients, there was a trend towards numerically more e-Stim treatments in those who achieved a pregnancy. In order to

128

confirm or refute differences in these two groups, Kaplan Meier's survival analyses were done. Based on these analyses, the average accumulated affect in the non-pregnant Ac group was 5.1 e-Stim treatments and 8.4 e-Stim treatments in the pregnant Ac group. This was statistically significantly different at the $p < 0.05$.

Conclusion: In traditional Chinese medicine the basic theory is that only when the body is balanced will it function at its optimal level. Acupuncture helps restore balance which results in a higher chance of achieving pregnancy. **In our study, we found that patients who received more than 8 e-Stim treatments appeared to have the maximum benefit for IVF outcomes: pregnancy ($p < 0.05$).** In our study, we also reviewed the independent effects of the Paulus protocol, however due to small numbers; we could not perform the analyses. In the IVF center included in this study, patients receive Valium (diazepam) to reduce smooth muscle contractility.

This treatment may provide all that is needed to reduce uterine contractility and therefore the additional impact of Ac at the pre and post transfer (Paulus protocol) may well be masked by the medication. More study of these and other treatments must be done. We are currently investigating the role of Ac in stress hormone circulating levels.

Effect of acupuncture on the pregnancy rate in embryo transfer and mechanisms: A randomized and controlled study

Zhang M et al, Chin Acup and Moxabustion 2003, Jan 23 (1): 3 - 5

A randomized, controlled, double-blind, cross-over study evaluating acupuncture as an adjunct to IVF Chinese Acupuncture and Moxabustion

210 IVF patients were randomly placed in groups that received real acupuncture or placebo or no treatment on the day of embryo transfer.

The pregnancy rate was significantly higher in the group who received real acupuncture. Additionally this trial showed that the women who received real acupuncture had fewer uterine cont ractions after the transfer.

Abstract

Objective To observe the effect of acupuncture on the pregnancy rate in assisted reproduction therapy such as in-vitro-fertilization (IVF) and intracytoplasmic spermatozoen injection (ICSI), and mechanisms.

Methods 210 cases undergoing IVF or ICSI were divided randomly into three groups: acupuncture treatment group, placebo group and control group. The acupuncture treatment group and the placebo group were treated respectively with body acupuncture and placebo acupuncture before and after embryo transfer, and in the control group embryos were transferred without any supportive therapy. Contraction frequency of the uterine junctional zone and the pregnancy rate were observed. Results The contraction frequency before embryo transfer was not significantly different among the three groups, but after embryo transfer in the acupuncture treatment group was lower than that in the placebo group and the control group, respectively. The pregnancy rate was 44.3% (31/70) in the acupuncture treatment group, and 27.1% (19/70) in the placebo group and 24.3% (17/70) in the control group. The pregnancy rate in the acupuncture treatment group was significantly higher than that in the placebo acupuncture group and the control group (P0.05).

Conclusion: **Acupuncture is a powerful tool for improving pregnancy rate after assisted reproduction therapy.**

Influence of acupuncture on the pregnancy rate in patients who undergo assisted reproduction therapy

Paulus W et al, Fertil Steril 2002 Vol 77, pg 721-724 Fertility and Sterility

Abstract

OBJECTIVE: To evaluate the effect of acupuncture on the pregnancy rate in assisted reproduction therapy (ART) by comparing a group of patients receiving acupuncture treatment shortly before and after embryo transfer with a control group receiving no acupuncture.

DESIGN:Prospectiverandomizedstudy.35 SETTING:Fertilitycenter.

PATIENT(S): After giving informed consent, 160 patients who were undergoing ART and who had good quality embryos were divided into the following two groups through random selection: embryo transfer with acupuncture (n = 80) and embryo transfer without acupuncture (n = 80).

INTERVENTION(S): Acupuncture was performed in 80 patients 25 minutes before and after embryo transfer. In the control group, embryos were transferred without any supportive therapy. MAIN OUTCOME MEASURE(S): Clinical pregnancy was defined as the presence of a fetal sac during an ultrasound examination 6 weeks after embryo transfer.
RESULT(S): Clinical pregnancies were documented in 34 of 80 patients (42.5%) in the acupuncture group, whereas pregnancy rate was only 26.3% (21 out of 80 patients) in the control group.
CONCLUSION(S): Acupuncture seems to be a useful tool for improving pregnancy rate after ART.

Acupuncture and IVF Miscellaneous

Acupuncture on the day of embryo transfer: a randomized controlled trial of 635 patients. Kong S. Hughes A Medical Acupuncture. 21(3) (pp 179-182), 2009. Abstract

Background: In vitro fertilization (IVF) is a widely accepted method to treat infertility; however, the average success rate in the United States is only 40.2%. Acupuncture has been shown to increase blood flow to the uterus, so it is reasonable to project that it could aid the success rate of IVF. Objective: To compare 3 acupuncture methods to evaluate which method is most effective for IVF. Design, Setting, and Patients: A total of 52 IVF patients aged between 29 and 45 years (mean age, 38) were selected for this study. This study was conducted from 2004 to 2008 at Acupuncture and Chinese Medical Center, Ann Arbor, MI. Interventions: Patients were randomly assigned to receive traditional Chinese acupuncture (TCA) plus electro acupuncture (EA), TCA alone (control), or EA alone (second control). Main Outcome Measures: Comparisons of IVF effectiveness rates were made for each method. Results: All 3 acupuncture methods increased the success rate for IVF. There was a marked increase with the combination of TCA and EA (81.8% success-twice the US average for IVF alone) (P < .01). The success rates for the control groups TCA and EA were 64.3% and 62.5%, respectively (P > .05).

Conclusions: **Our study suggests that the combination of TCA and EA is a promising new technique for the treatment of infertility with a higher IVF success rate than that of TCA or EA alone.**

Acupuncture as an adjunct to in vitro fertilization: A randomized trial.

Kong S. Hughes A. Medical Acupuncture 2009;21:179-82.

A randomized controlled trial that compared three acupuncture methods to evaluate which method is most effective for IVF. A total of 52 IVF patients were randomly assigned to receive traditional Chinese acupuncture plus electro acupuncture, acupuncture alone (control), or electro acupuncture alone (second control). Comparisons of IVF effectiveness rates were made for each method. All three acupuncture methods increased the success rate for IVF, and there was a marked increase with the combination treatment (81.8% success, which is twice the US average for IVF alone; p<0.01). The success rates for the control groups were 64.3% with acupuncture and 62.5% with electro acupuncture (p>0.05). **The researchers concluded that their results suggest the combination of acupuncture and electro acupuncture is a promising new technique for the treatment of infertility with a higher IVF success rate than that of either treatment alone.**

Acupuncture intervention combined with assisted reproductive technology: Its different effects at different time points during the in vitro fertilization-embryo transfer course

Guo J. Li D. Zhang Q.-F.

Department of Traditional Chinese Medicine and Acupuncture, Peking University Third Hospital, Beijing 100191, China [in Chinese] Journal of Chinese Integrative Medicine. 6(12)(pp 1211- 1216), 2008.

Recently the combination of acupuncture with assisted reproductive technology (ART) to increase the outcomes of ART is being widely studied. In this article, the literatures concerning random controlled clinical trials since 2002 are reviewed and the designs of the trials, especially the timing of acupuncture, are evaluated. Over the past 5 years, the related clinical trials have primarily showed that acupuncture done immediately before and after embryo transfer might increase the assisted reproduction rates, but still requiring further high quality trials with large samples; in addition, different stimulation modes could produce different result, and so far there has not been a consensus as to the optimal time-point for the acupuncture intervention during the in vitro fertilization-embryo transfer (IVF-ET) course. Since the effects of acupuncture change with women's endocrine cycles, it is important and possible to make a breakthrough in ART outcomes if acupuncture is performed at a suitable time point during the cycle of IVF/ET combined with ART.

In vitro fertilization and acupuncture: clinical efficacy and mechanistic basis.

Anderson BJ, Haimovici F, Ginsburg ES, Schust DJ, Wayne PM. Pacific College of Oriental Medicine, New York, USA. Altern Ther Health Med. 2007 May-Jun;13(3):38-48.

OBJECTIVE: To provide an overview of the use of acupuncture as an adjunct therapy for in vitro fertilization (IVF), including an evidence-based evaluation of its efficacy and safety and an examination of possible mechanisms of action. DESIGN: Literature review using PubMed, the Science Citation Index, The Cochrane Library (Database of Systematic Reviews and Central Register of Controlled Trials), the New England School of Acupuncture library databases, and a cross-referencing of published data, personal libraries, and Chinese medicine textbooks. RESULTS: Limited but supportive evidence from clinical trials and case series suggests that acupuncture may improve the success rate of IVF and the quality of life of patients undergoing IVF and that it is a safe adjunct therapy. However, this conclusion should be interpreted with caution because most studies reviewed had design limitations, and the acupuncture interventions employed often were not consistent with traditional Chinese medical principles. The reviewed literature suggests 4 possible mechanisms by which acupuncture could improve the outcome of IVF: modulating neuroendocrinological factors; increasing blood flow to the uterus and ovaries; modulating cytokines; and reducing stress, anxiety, and depression.

CONCLUSIONS: **More high-quality randomized, controlled trials incorporating placebo acupuncture controls, authentic acupuncture interventions, and a range of outcome measures representative of both clinical outcomes and putative mechanistic processes are required to better assess the efficacy of acupuncture as an adjunct for IVF.**

Acupuncture and wellbeing of IVF patients

An assessment of the demand and importance of acupuncture to patients of a fertility clinic during investigations and treatment Hinks J and Coulson C, Hum Fert 2010 Vol 13, S1 Pg 3-21 Human Fertility

These authors working in a fertility clinic in the UK surveyed 200 patients who attended the clinic in August 2009. They discovered that there was a clear demand for acupuncture and that acupuncture may be valuable to improve the general well-being of women during infertility investigations and treatments. They also felt that patient resilience may be increased by the use of acupuncture alongside their IVF treatment such that patients would persevere with increased numbers of ART (Assisted Reproductive Technologies) cycles, thereby increasing their ultimate chance of a successful pregnancy.

An assessment of the demand and importance of acupuncture to patients of a fertility clinic during investigations and treatment

Julie Hinks & Catherine Coulson

North Bristol NHS Trust, Bristol, United Kingdom

Introduction. Despite a lack of studies clearly demonstrating clinical efficacy complementary medicine is frequently used by couples undergoing infertility treatment

(Coulson 2005). In Bristol, acupuncture has become very popular among patients undergoing infertility treatment, thus this study sought to quantify this and examine the reasons why patients choose acupuncture.

Methods. Two hundred questionnaires were given to patients who attended the Bristol Centre for Reproductive Medicine (BCRM) for investigation or treatment of infertility in August 2009. Patients were asked to complete the questionnaire while waiting to see their doctor or nurse and 194 responses were returned. The questionnaires asked if patients had or wished to have acupuncture or other complementary medicine, and to indicate on a scale of one to ten (10 being the best) the relative importance of acupuncture in comparison to values such as pregnancy rates and continuity of care.

Results. Out of 58 respondents who use complementary medicine, 43 used acupuncture. 40 respondents use acupuncture regularly and 17 of those lived outside of Bristol. A further 52 respondents had considered using acupuncture. In terms of very high importance (score of 10) 135 respondents felt pregnancy rates scored 10, 84 felt having the same doctor scored 10, 71 scored 10 for having the same nurse, 31 felt in house acupuncture scored 10 and 21 scored 10 65 for other complementary medicine. Overall, 43 respondents felt acupuncture should be available at Bristol Centre for Reproductive Medicine. Thirty-four respondents gave more importance to acupuncture than seeing the same doctor or nurse, and 32 deemed it equally important. In addition, 29 patients scored acupuncture as equally important to pregnancy rates and 5 scored acupuncture higher than pregnancy rates.

Discussion: Previous unpublished work at BCRM showed that 85% of the patients found the named nurse system important as a coping mechanism to support them by providing continuity of care through stressful treatment. The responses to the questionnaires indicate a clear demand for acupuncture and suggest that acupuncture may be valuable to improve the general wellbeing of women during infertility investigations and treatments. If acupuncture provides an effective coping mechanism, this could support patients to persevere with increased numbers of ART(Assisted Reproductive Technologies) cycles, thereby increasing their ultimate chance of a successful pregnancy.

Building resilience: An exploration of women's perceptions of the use of acupuncture as an adjunct to IVF

De Lacey S, Smith C and Paterson C, BMC Complementary and Alternative Medicine 2009, 9:50

Resilience is an interesting and important concept when applied to couples doing IVF.

Studies of acupuncture involving women dealing with chronic health issues have shown that women experienced relief of presenting symptoms but also increases in energy, increase in relaxation and calmness, reduction in the reliance of prescription drugs (such as analgesics), quicker healing from surgery and increased self-awareness and wellbeing. Such effects indicate a reduction of stress that in turn may diminish the number of treatment cycles needed for pregnancy to occur. But further, reducing the number of cycles a woman must undertake to reach her goal of motherhood reduces the overall cost of IVF.

Abstract Background

In Vitro Fertilization (IVF) is now an accepted and effective treatment for infertility, however IVF is acknowledged as contributing to, rather than lessening, the overall psychosocial effects of infertility. Psychological and counseling interventions have previously been widely recommended in parallel with infertility treatments but whilst in many jurisdictions counseling is recommended or mandatory, it may not be widely used. Acupuncture is increasingly used as an adjunct to IVF, in this preliminary study we sought to investigate the experience of infertile women who had used acupuncture to improve their fertility.

Methods

A sample of 20 women was drawn from a cohort of women who had attended for a minimum of four acupuncture sessions in the practices of two acupuncturists in South Australia. Eight women were interviewed using a semi-structured questionnaire. Six had sought acupuncture during IVF treatment and two had begun acupuncture to enhance their fertility and had later progressed to IVF. Descriptive content analysis was employed to analyze the data.

Results

Four major categories of perceptions about acupuncture in relation to reproductive health were identified: (a) Awareness of, and perceived benefits of acupuncture; (b) perceptions of the body and the impact of acupuncture upon it; (c) perceptions of stress and the impact of acupuncture on resilience; and (d) perceptions of the intersection of medical treatment and acupuncture.

Conclusion: This preliminary exploration, whilst confined to a small sample of women, confirms that acupuncture is indeed perceived by infertile women to have an impact to their health. All findings outlined here are reported cautiously because they are limited by the size of the sample. They suggest that further studies of acupuncture as an adjunct to IVF should systematically explore the issues of wellbeing, anxiety, personal and social resilience and women's identity in relation to sexuality and reproduction.http://www.biomedcentral.com/ 1472-6882/9/50

The relationship between perceived stress, acupuncture, and pregnancy rates among IVF patients: A pilot study

Balk J et al, Complementary Therapies in Clinical Practice, Online 24 December 2009

Complementary Therapies in Clinical Practice

These investigators aimed to determine if acupuncture affects the levels of perceived stress at the time of embryo transfer, and whether either acupuncture or changes in stress levels play a role int he success rate in IVF. The patients who received acupuncture in this study had both higher rates of pregnancy, and lower levels of stress both before and after embryo transfer. They postulated that reducing stress at the time of embryo transfer could result in less vasoconstriction and improved uterine receptivity.

Abstract

The aim of this paper was to determine the effect of acupuncture on perceived stress levels in women on the day of embryo transfer (ET), and to determine if perceived stress levels at embryo transfer correlated with pregnancy rates. The study was an observational, prospective, cohort study based at the University IVF center.

Patient(s): 57 infertile patients undergoing IVF or IVF/ICSI. Interventions(s): Patients were undergoing Embryo Transfer with or without acupuncture as part of their standard clinical care.

Conclusion: **Acupuncture is an effective and low intensity procedure for increasing women's resilience in the repetitive and stress-inducing time of pregnancy attempts, with or without medical treatment. The instrumental role of the acupuncture therapist in increasing resilience is a finding that has not emerged in previous studies and has implications for patient management.**

Changes in serum cortisol and prolactin associated with acupuncture during controlled ovarian hyperstimulation in women undergoing in vitro fertilization–embryo transfer treatment

Magarelli, PC, D Cridennda, M Cohen. Fertil Steril. 2009 Dec;92(6): 1870-9 Fertility and Sterility

A number of women going through IVF were given acupuncture to increase blood flow through the uterine arteries in the immediate weeks before egg collection. The researchers found that the women who had acupuncture showed beneficial changes in serum levels of stress hormones compared to the control group of women who did not have acupuncture. The acupuncture treatments appear to normalize levels of cortisol and prolactin, which have been artificially depressed by the IVF drugs. This may have implications for both egg quality and implantation. In addition the pregnancy and live birth rate was significantly higher in the acupuncture group.

Abstract

Objective: To determine whether changes in serum cortisol (CORT) and PRL are affected by acupuncture (Ac) in Ac-treated IVF patients.

Design: Prospective cohort clinical study.

Setting: Private practice reproductive endocrinology and infertility clinic and private practice acupuncture consortium. Main outcome measure(s): Perceive Stress Scale scores, pregnancy rates.

Result(s): **women who received this acupuncture regimen achieved pregnancy 64.7%, whereas those without acupuncture achieved pregnancy 42.5%.** When stratified by donor recipient status, only non-donor recipients potentially had an improvement with acupuncture (35.5% without acupuncture vs. 55.6% with acupuncture). Those who received this acupuncture regimen had lower stress scores both pre-ET and post-ET compared to those who did not. Those with decreased their perceived stress scores compared to baseline had higher pregnancy rates than those who did not demonstrate this decrease, regardless of acupuncture status.

Conclusions(s): **The acupuncture regimen was associated with less stress both before and after embryo transfer, and it possibly improved pregnancy rates. Lower perceived stress at the time of embryo transfer may play a role in an improved pregnancy rate.**

Understanding Women's views towards the use of Acupuncture While Undergoing IVF Treatment.

Smith C and De Lacey S, 2008 In press FSA conference 2008

This qualitative study found that most women who had acupuncture as an adjunct to IVF treatment reported increased wellbeing, reduced anxiety and an increase in capacity to cope with the stresses of IVF and infertility treatments.

Abstract

Aim: There is interest in the use of acupuncture as an adjunct to fertility treatment. This study aimed to examine women's attitudes and beliefs in relation to the use of acupuncture for enhancing fertility or as an adjunct to ART.

Results: Participants all expressed confidence in the ability of acupuncture to contribute to their reproductive decision in a positive way. They described acupuncture as an adjunct to pregnancy attempts that was positive since it gave them a sense of control and a strategy for improving their chances. Patient(s): Sixty-seven reproductive-age infertile women undergoing IVF.

Intervention(s): Blood samples were obtained from all consenting new infertility patients and serum CORT and serum PRL were obtained prospectively. Patients were grouped as controls (IVF with no Ac) and treated (IVF with Ac) according to acupuncture protocols derived from randomized controlled trials.

Main Outcome Measure(s): Serum levels of CORT and PRL were measured and synchronized with medication stimulation days of the IVF cycle (e.g., day 2 of stimulation, day 3, etc.). Reproductive outcomes were collected according to Society for Assisted Reproductive Technology protocols, and results were compared between controls and those patients treated with Ac.

Result(s): CORT levels in Ac group were significantly higher on IVF medication days 7, 8, 9, 11, 12, and 13 compared with controls. PRL levels in the Ac group were significantly higher on IVF medication days 5, 6, 7, and 8 compared with controls.

Conclusion(s): **In this study, there appears to be a beneficial regulation of CORT and PRL in the Ac group during the medication phase of the IVF treatment.**

Effects of electro acupuncture on in vitro fertilization-embryo transfer (IVF- ET) of patients with poor ovarian response.

Chen J et al [Chinese] Zhongguo Zhenjiu 2009;29:775-9

A randomized controlled trial to observe the effect of electro acupuncture therapy on oocyte quality and pregnancy outcome of 60 patients with poor ovarian response or decreased reserve in the course of in vitro fertilization (IVF). The levels of serum estradiol, fertilization rate, oocyte maturation rate, good quality embryos rate, and implantation rate in the acupuncture group were superior to those in the control group on the day of human Chorionic Gonadotropin (hCG) injection (all $p < 0.05$). Also, the levels of stem cell factor in follicular fluid and serum in the acupuncture group were significantly higher than those in the control group (both $p < 0.05$). The researchers concluded that electro acupuncture therapy has a good clinical effect for IVF patients with poor ovarian reserve, and can improve oocyte quality and pregnancy outcome

Our Fertility Plan

Important Labs & Phone Numbers:

Medications & Supplements Currently Taking:

Treatments Undergone:

Practitioner Notes Regarding Our Plan (To Be Shared With My Other Fertility Specialists):

About the Author

Farrar V. Duro, DOM, FABORM, Dipl. Ac. is a licensed Acupuncture Physician and Fellow of the American Board of Oriental Reproductive Medicine (ABORM) specializing in the treatment of infertility with acupuncture and Chinese herbal medicine. She served as the first staff acupuncturist at the UHealth Fertility Center at the University of Miami in Miami, Florida and has been in private practice at Florida Complete Wellness since 2001.

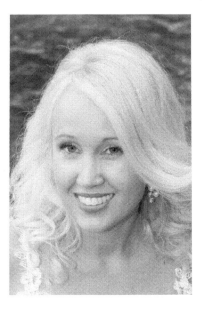

Farrar Duro holds a past faculty position at her alma mater, the Florida College of Integrative Medicine and is a professional member of the Florida State Oriental Medical Association, RESOLVE (the National Infertility Association), and the American Society for Reproductive Medicine (ASRM).

After overcoming her own struggles with PCOS using a combination of Traditional Chinese Medicine and other natural methods, she has felt tremendous joy in sharing her methods with other women.

Dr. Duro has since specialized in the treatment of PCOS, infertility and hormonal imbalances with acupuncture and Chinese herbal medicine since 2004 and has a passion for women's health and wellness.

This path led her to pursue advanced pregnancy training in the Arvigo Techniques of Maya Abdominal Therapy and publication of her first book, *The Smart Couple's Guide to Getting Pregnant, An Integrated Approach* in 2015.

A board-certified acupuncture physician, Dr. Duro graduated from the Florida College of Integrative Medicine and performed her post-graduate training at Shandong University of TCM in Shandong, China. She holds regular speaking engagements at local universities, hospitals and IVF centers to advocate for a better understanding of integrative women's health between patients, doctors and other complementary healthcare providers. To learn more, go to www.floridacompletewellness.com.